# CBT for Long-Term Conditions and Medically Unexplained Symptoms

*CBT for Long-Term Conditions and Medically Unexplained Symptoms* describes how cognitive behavioural therapy (CBT) can be used to treat anxiety and depression with a co-morbid long-term physical health condition (LTC) or medically unexplained symptoms (MUS).

The book teaches cognitive behavioural therapists and other clinicians to help patients deal with the psychological aspects of physical symptoms, whatever their cause. It is divided into three parts, beginning with core skills for working with people with LTC and MUS. This includes assessment, formulation and goal setting. Part II focuses on CBT for LTC and includes chapters on low-intensity interventions, working with depression and anxiety using protocols, and a consideration of an identity and strengths-based approach to working with LTC. The final part provides details of a formulation-driven approach to working with MUS, broken down into individual chapters on working with behaviours, cognitions and emotions.

With numerous case examples, the book provides accessible and practical guidance for mental health professionals, particularly CBT practitioners, working with anyone with long-term conditions or MUS.

**Philip Kinsella** is a CBT practitioner specialising in psychological medicine, and a lecturer in CBT at Nottingham university training IAPT practitioners. He is the co-author of *Cognitive Behavioural Therapy for Mental Health Workers* and author of *Cognitive Behavioural Therapy for Chronic Fatigue Syndrome*.

**Dr Helen Moya** is a CBT practitioner and Chartered Psychologist. She currently works in a UK IAPT service and has her own private practice. Previously the Course Director of a CBT training programme at the University of Nottingham, she has an academic background rooted in psychology and mental health.

# CBT for Long-Term Conditions and Medically Unexplained Symptoms

A Practitioner's Guide

Philip Kinsella and Helen Moya

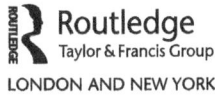
Routledge
Taylor & Francis Group

LONDON AND NEW YORK

First published 2022
by Routledge
2 Park Square, Milton Park, Abingdon, Oxon OX14 4RN

and by Routledge
605 Third Avenue, New York, NY 10158

*Routledge is an imprint of the Taylor & Francis Group, an informa business*

© 2022 Philip Kinsella and Helen Moya

The right of Philip Kinsella and Helen Moya to be identified as authors of this work has been asserted by them in accordance with sections 77 and 78 of the Copyright, Designs and Patents Act 1988.

*British Library Cataloguing-in-Publication Data*
A catalogue record for this book is available from the British Library

*Library of Congress Cataloging-in-Publication Data*
Names: Kinsella, Philip, author. | Moya, Helen, author.
Title: CBT for long-term conditions and medically unexplained symptoms : a practitioner's guide / Philip Kinsella and Helen Moya.
Description: Milton Park, Abingdon, Oxon New York, NY : Routledge, 2022. | Includes bibliographical references and index.
Identifiers: LCCN 2021024521 (print) | LCCN 2021024522 (ebook) | ISBN 9780367424893 (hardback) | ISBN 9780367424879 (paperback) | ISBN 9780367824433 (ebook)
Subjects: LCSH: Long-term care of the sick. | Cognitive therapy.
Classification: LCC RT120.L64 K56 2022 (print) | LCC RT120.L64 (ebook) | DDC 362.16—dc23
LC record available at https://lccn.loc.gov/2021024521
LC ebook record available at https://lccn.loc.gov/2021024522

ISBN: 978-0-367-42489-3 (hbk)
ISBN: 978-0-367-42487-9 (pbk)
ISBN: 978-0-367-82443-3 (ebk)

DOI: 10.4324/9780367824433

Typeset in Times New Roman
by Apex CoVantage, LLC

PK dedication: to my wife Hazel, for her kindness and support.

HM dedication: I dedicate this book to my family, who have always supported me through all my endeavours and adventures.

# Contents

# Figures and Tables

## Figures

## Tables

# Introduction

This book describes how to use cognitive behavioural therapy (CBT) for people with a co-morbid long-term physical health condition (LTC), or medically unexplained symptoms (MUS), with depression or anxiety. The material comprises a blend of the available research evidence, NHS guidelines and the experience of the authors who both have expertise in working with these presentations. Philip Kinsella has worked as a cognitive behavioural therapist for over 25 years, specialising in LTC and MUS within a department of psychological medicine in a UK-based medical training hospital. He is also an academic and trains cognitive behavioural therapists and Helen Moya was one of his students in 2009. Since this time, they have worked together both in the same clinical setting and as fellow academics and trainers on the high-intensity CBT course at the University of Nottingham. More recently, Helen Moya has returned to full-time clinical practice in an Improving Access to Psychological Therapies (IAPT) service (primary care psychological therapy service in England) where she has treated people with LTC and MUS in a much shorter time-limited manner.

The book is aimed at qualified cognitive behavioural therapists who have basic training in CBT for adults with depression or anxiety. Knowledge and skills in working with a range of anxiety disorders and depression will be assumed. Unlike most mental health conditions, where there is substantial research evidence as to the effectiveness of specific CBT protocols, psychological therapies for LTC and MUS remain an area that lacks a broad evidence base. There is a general message in the book that disorder-specific CBT protocols can be used, and adapted if necessary, when working with people with LTC. For MUS the complexity of the presentations, and rigidity of beliefs, makes a formulation-driven transdiagnostic approach more fruitful. This is in line with current available evidence, which is presented throughout.

The current context of stepped care in the UK (NICE, 2009) demands an understanding of the levels of psychological interventions for treating depression in the presence of a physical health condition. This goes from threshold and mild symptoms of depression, suitable for Step 2 or low-intensity interventions normally delivered by psychological well-being practitioners (PWPs) in IAPT services. Step 3 relates to moderate-to-severe symptoms of depression, which are delivered

DOI: 10.4324/9780367824433-1

by trained cognitive behavioural therapists accredited by the British Association for Behavioural and Cognitive Psychotherapies (BABCP). For more complex presentations Step 4 interventions in specialist secondary and tertiary care services, such as psychological medicine and other adult mental health services, can be delivered. Much of this book is aimed primarily at a Steps 3 and 4 approach, but Chapter 4 is dedicated to a Step 2 approach to psychological interventions for people with LTC or MUS.

The book is divided into three parts, beginning with core skills for working with people with LTC and MUS. This includes assessment, formulation and goal setting. Part II focuses on CBT for LTC and includes chapters on low-intensity interventions, working with depression and anxiety using protocols, and a consideration of identity and strengths-based approach to working with LTC. The final section provides details of a formulation-driven approach to working with MUS, broken down into individual chapters on working with behaviours, cognitions and emotions. It also includes a reflective chapter on the lived experience of having MUS by one of the authors (Helen Moya) and finishes with a consideration of how we can help people who may fear recovery.

The book was written during the onset and continuation of the Covid-19 pandemic in 2020. The authors recognise that it is affecting mental health, and the after-effects of the virus are likely to impact on many people in the form of what has become known as Long Covid, to an extent that is not known, and we discuss this in Chapter 1. A related issue to the current context of the pandemic is the change in working practices of cognitive behavioural therapists from face-to-face live therapy to remote working. This includes telephone, video and internet-based platforms. The approaches presented in the book are largely based on traditional face-to-face CBT but the chapter on low-intensity CBT details many methods and techniques that lend themselves to remote working.

# Part I

# Core skills to treat long-term medical conditions, and medically unexplained symptoms

# Chapter 1

# Core skills in understanding and helping this patient group

## Why there is a need for a psychological approach in this area

Around 27 per cent of the English population have one or more long-term health conditions, including diabetes, arthritis, asthma and various cardiovascular diseases. To these can be added conditions such as HIV/AIDs and certain cancers, which are increasingly regarded as long-term conditions, rather than fatal illnesses. Thirty per cent of people with LTCs will experience a mental health problem (Department of Health, 2015). There is evidence for a particularly close association between mental health problems and specific health conditions, namely cardiovascular diseases, diabetes, chronic obstructive pulmonary disease (COPD), musculoskeletal disorders, asthma, arthritis, cancer and HIV/AIDs (Sederer, Dermen, Carruthers & Wall, 2016). Mental disorders can also precipitate and influence physical problems: depression increases the risk for onset of coronary artery disease and ischaemic heart disease 0.5- to 2-fold (Benton, Staab & Evans, 2007). Chronic stress has a direct impact on the cardiovascular, nervous and immune systems, leading to increased vulnerability to a range of diseases (Contrada & Baum, 2010). As a result of these associations, people with mental health problems are two to four times more likely to die prematurely (Eaton et al., 2008).

As a result of this situation, in England, IAPT services are being expanding to the LTC/MUS area, services are being commissioned and staff are being trained. Pathways are being developed, with the recommendation that 75% of patients should be seen within 6 weeks, and 95% within 18 weeks of referral and 50% should move to recovery. Patients should be provided with ease of access, the most effective, least intrusive service and trained and competent therapists, and treatment should be informed by patient choice and the NICE guidelines (National Collaboration Centre, 2018). It is suggested that the ideal workforce should be 10% health or clinical psychologists, 60% 'high intensity' practitioners (delivering CBT or NICE recommended therapies) and 30% psychological wellbeing practitioners (PWPs). It is recommended that patients are offered help from the least intrusive and most effective NICE recommended therapy first. Therefore, a patient could be offered low-intensity work from a PWP, stepping up to high intensity

DOI: 10.4324/9780367824433-3

(including CBT), or, from a psychologist or senior therapist located in IAPT or elsewhere if available and accessible: how this is decided would be based on the severity, chronicity and complexity of the mental and physical health problem, any relevant environmental factors, degree of disability and complexity of the medical condition. What are the specific groups of patients that we are describing?

## Patients with a long-term health condition

Looking in detail at the three main groups of patients, the first group are the patients who have a *long-term (health) condition* (also known as a chronic illness), such as rheumatoid arthritis or diabetes, and who develop an anxiety or depressive disorder. An example is Alice, who has been diagnosed with Parkinson's disease some years ago, and is deteriorating in her functioning, she suffers from tremors and spasms. She has a diagnosis of depression, and her thoughts are 'I'm getting worse, I'm a burden, I don't have much of a life.' At times she is more active, and she reads and does housework with difficulty, with the help of her partner; other times she is more withdrawn and does little.

(A question arises as to how much the psychological therapist needs to understand the medical condition that the person is suffering from. Our experience is that one does need to have a reasonable knowledge of the conditions, but is not realistic or necessary to be an expert. Common medical problems met, as described in the Table 1.1, are based on information on the NHS website, which provides a basic level of knowledge for the therapist).

*Table 1.1* Long-term conditions (the patient may have one of these and develop anxiety/depression)

| Conditions | Description |
| --- | --- |
| Cancer | Cells in a specific part of the body grow and reproduce abnormally, and when the cancer spreads to other areas, this is called metastasis. The most common cancers are breast, lung, prostate and bowel. One in 3 people will develop this in their lifetime. |
| Neurological problems | A common problem seen is multiple sclerosis; symptoms are problems with vision, arm or leg movement, sensation or balance. It usually occurs in people in their 20s–30s, and is 2–3 times more in women. There is no cure, but it can be helped by medications. |
| | Parkinson's disease is a condition in which parts of the brain become progressively damaged over the years, and the typical symptoms are tremor, slow movement and stiff muscles. |
| Diabetes | This illness is of two types: in type 1, the immune system destroys the cells that produce insulin. In the more common type 2 (90% of adult sufferers), usually the body does not produce enough insulin. The patient needs to take injections of insulin or adjust their lifestyle and diet. |

| Conditions | Description |
| --- | --- |
| Arthritis | There is pain and inflammation in a joint; osteoarthritis is the most common type. It develops in people who are over 40, more commonly in women and people with a family history of the disorder: the most common joints affected are hands, spine, knees and hips. Rheumatoid arthritis is less common, and women are 3 times more affected. |
| Heart disease | The most common manifestations are angina, heart attacks and heart failure. Angina is reduced blood flow to the heart causing chest pain. Heart attacks (Myocardial Infarctions) are serious conditions in which the blood supply to the heart is blocked, usually by a blood clot; this can damage the heart muscle and be life threatening. Heart failure is a long-term condition, where the heart is not working properly, with symptoms of tiredness, breathlessness and swollen legs. |
| Renal conditions | The kidneys filter the blood, and in kidney failure they don't work as well as they could. Symptoms can range from nothing, to tiredness, swollen ankles/feet, breathlessness and feeling sick. |
| Respiratory conditions | Chronic obstructive pulmonary disease (COPD) is the name for a group of lung conditions that cause breathing difficulties, which tend to get worse over time. Main symptoms are breathlessness, persistent cough, frequent chest infections and wheezing. Asthma is a common lung condition that causes breathing difficulties. The symptoms are wheezing, tight chest, breathlessness and coughing. |

## Adjustment disorder

Another thing to consider is the possibility that the patient is suffering from an adjustment disorder. This is described in the Diagnostic and Statistical manual of Mental disorder (American Psychiatric Association, 2013) as the development of emotional or behavioural symptoms in response to a stressor occurring within three months from the onset of the stressor. Their response can be anxiety, depression or a mixture, and it is out of proportion to the intensity of the stressor, and causes significant impairment. The presentation here is of a patient who would not meet the diagnostic criteria for clinical depression or an actual anxiety disorder. Typically, the patient receives a diagnosis of a medical condition, possibly not of the more severe type, or develops symptoms, and struggles to cope with this for various reasons. It is often a person who is quite well resourced and normally able to cope with things. We would observe that they are demoralised, they may have become excessively avoidant, they may not be looking after their health very well and they may be having negative thoughts such as 'I can't cope with this' and 'I am a failure'. Simply allowing patients to tell their story and allow for emotional processing and expression is helpful, and CBT here is relatively simple: tackling avoidance behaviours, challenging day-to-day negative thoughts and building on the patient's strengths and resources. We would expect this to be a relatively short piece of work with a good outcome.

## Patients with medically unexplained symptoms

The next group seen are the patients who have *medically unexplained symptoms:* this means that their symptoms of, for example, pain or fatigue have not been explained by standard medical investigations (or sometimes the symptoms seem disproportionate to the level of pathology that has been medically detected). For example, Julie describes her main problem as feeling tired, weak in her legs, with strange sensations and dizziness. Despite investigations, no medical reasons for these symptoms have been found, which reassured her as she was previously worried that she had multiple sclerosis. She believes she cannot do as much as she used to do, or her muscles will get more painful, so she avoids activity to prevent worsening the symptoms. She now accepts the symptoms are stress related. The onset was two years prior; she had lots of responsibility, and was working long days; one of her managers at work was difficult and set unrealistic targets for the work, which was a major source of stress. She then attended her general practitioner (GP) who said that the symptoms would settle down, and she had physiotherapy.

Medical doctors, psychiatrists and the patients themselves have different labels for these problems, and this table may help the reader.

*Table 1.2* Common medically unexplained symptoms and diagnostic labels by medical speciality

| Speciality | Common medically unexplained symptoms | Typical diagnostic labels |
|---|---|---|
| Psychiatry | Varies | Somatoform disorder, somatisation disorder, somatic syndrome disorder health anxiety |
| Gastroenterology | Abdominal pain; diarrhoea; bloating; constipation; excessive flatulence | Irritable bowel syndrome; non-ulcer dyspepsia |
| Cardiology | Chest pain; palpitations; fainting | Non-cardiac chest pain, atypical chest pain |
| Neurology | Walking and gait disturbance; headaches; seizures; sensory disturbance | Non-epileptic attack disorder; Pseudo-seizures, conversion disorder, functional neurological disorder |
| Rheumatology | Joint pain; fatigue | Fibromyalgia |

| Speciality | Common medically unexplained symptoms | Typical diagnostic labels |
|---|---|---|
| Infectious diseases | Fatigue; headaches; poor concentration; joint pain | Chronic (post-viral) fatigue syndrome (aka myalgic encephalomyelitis) |
| Dentistry | Facial pain; headaches; tinnitus | Atypical facial pain; Temporomandibular joint disorder |
| Ear, nose and throat | Lump in throat; breathing problems; loss of voice or speaking difficulties | Globus syndrome; functional voice loss; psychogenic voice disorder |
| Allergy | Fatigue; burning eyes; breathlessness; poor concentration; weakness; dizziness | Multiple chemical sensitivity |
| Respiratory medicine | Breathlessness; rapid breathing | Hyperventilation syndrome |
| Gynaecology | Pelvic pain; pain during sex; dysmenorrhea; painful urination; urinary retention | Chronic pelvic pain |
| Military medicine | Fatigue; headaches; muscle pains; neurological symptoms; poor concentration | Gulf war syndrome |

Source: From Brown (2004)

## Patients with health anxiety

The third group are patients who have *health anxiety* (sometimes called 'illness anxiety disorder' or hypochondriasis); these patients have physical symptoms that they worry about excessively, and think are likely to be dangerous or fatal. These health anxiety patients sometimes have health anxiety as a diagnosis, sometimes they have health anxiety as part of an actual long-term condition or medically unexplained symptom, so they can overlap as seen as follows:

So, these three groups of patients have some things in common, and some differences, in common they have physical symptoms that they are struggling with. In LTC the patients have serious and possibly life-threatening symptoms that make it hard to live a full life, and these may have contributed to an episode of anxiety or depression. With MUS psychological processes are generating physical symptoms, and these processes like stress and avoidance need to be understood and tackled. In health anxiety the patients may or may not have an actual medical condition, but they are misinterpreting the symptoms as being more dangerous than they are.

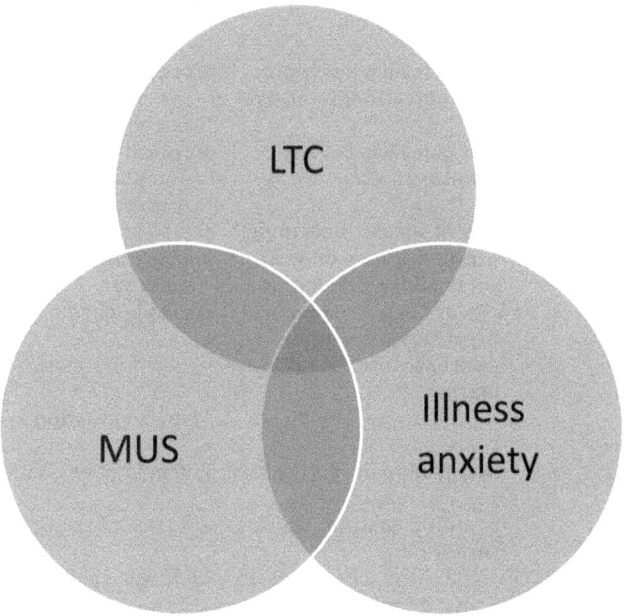

*Figure 1.1* Overlap of problems

## Covid-19

Relatively high rates of anxiety, depression, post-traumatic stress disorder, psychological distress and stress were reported in the general population during the Covid-19 pandemic in eight countries. Common risk factors associated with mental distress during the Covid-19 pandemic include female gender, younger age group (≤40 years), presence of chronic/psychiatric illnesses, unemployment, student status and frequent exposure to social media/news concerning Covid-19 (Xiong et al., 2020). Characteristics of the pandemic (e.g. physical risks, daily disruptions, uncertainty, social isolation, financial loss, the long and widespread nature and poor availability of protections) are known to affect mental health Gruber et al. (2020).

Patients with long-term conditions, for example respiratory illness and diabetes, have been hard hit, many losing their lives. People who tend to worry about their health will do so more whilst the virus is at large; there is already some evidence of an increase in health anxiety, and association with online reassurance seeking Jungmann and Witthöft (2020). The isolation and lack of valuable activities are likely to impact on people's mood. Long Covid-19 patients may have problems with fatigue and other symptoms. There is some initial research (not peer reviewed at the time of writing) on medically unexplained symptoms showing an increased attendance of these patients at the emergency department (Daniels, Ridwan, Barnard, Amanullah & Hayhurst, 2021). However, we do think that the interventions described in this book still hold true, and do not need modification because of the pandemic, or we note where modifications could be made under each disorder. If there is a significant increase in cases, low-intensity mass interventions may be helpful.

## Evidence for effectiveness of CBT

In a Cochrane review of treatments for MUS (Van Dessel et al., 2014) CBT delivered by specially trained therapists is more effective than usual care, but effect sizes are small, but durable at one year. CBT is no more effective than enhanced care provided by the person's doctor (GP) (Van Dessel et al., 2014). The methodology of the review has been criticised as underestimating the impact of CBT because of inclusion criteria (Schröder, Sharpe & Fink, 2015). The Cochrane review did not support the effectiveness of psychodynamic, behavioural therapy or psychodynamic therapy based on a small number of studies. A more recent meta-analysis (Liu, Gill, Teodorczuk, Li & Sun, 2018) had comparable results: suggesting that CBT is moderately efficacious for somatoform disorders and MUS in reducing somatic symptoms, anxiety symptoms, depressive symptoms and improving physical functioning. The effects of CBT on alleviating somatic symptoms, anxiety and depressive symptoms do persist at follow-up.

Regarding depression and anxiety in long-term health conditions, CBT has some evidence (Clarke & Currie, 2009) in particular there is evidence that CBT is 'modestly effective' for depression and anxiety in patients with heart disease, diabetes, range of cancers and arthritis. We can therefore conclude that CBT is a legitimate treatment for these problems with fairly modest effects.

## Are medications or diets worth considering?

In terms of medication for somatoform disorders in adults (Kleinstäuber et al., 2015), there is no difference in efficacy between tricyclic antidepressants and placebo on the severity of symptoms: new-generation antidepressants such as selective serotonin reuptake inhibitors (SSRIs) and serotonin and norepinephrine reuptake inhibitors (SNRIs) may have a moderate effect on symptom severity versus placebo; and natural products, for example herbal remedies such as St John's wort, may reduce the severity of symptoms and other secondary outcomes compared with placebo. Of course, antidepressants could be used for depression, as with people who do not have a long-term condition, and one review sees them as 'modestly effective' (Clarke & Currie, 2009). Drug treatments are being trialled for irritable bowel syndrome (IBS), and the low FODMAP diet (effectively reducing apples, pears, wheat, onion, legumes, stone fruit, artificial sweeteners and lactose) has an evidence base of effectiveness (Marsh, Eslick & Eslick, 2016).

## What are the core CBT and additional skills with this group?

The core CBT skills are collaboration, Socratic questioning and guided discovery, building a formulation, setting goals and agreeing homework. If we look at these, in turn, collaboration is important, particularly listening carefully to the patient's story and acknowledging the distress; and strong collaboration is required in the setting of goals, in particular the balance between acceptance and change. Guided discovery and Socratic questioning will help them gently consider different perspectives: it's important with this group to help them think about whether their response to illness is normal, a problem with adjustment or that they have descended into depression. Another area is to help them think about, particularly in MUS, how psychological and stress factors can contribute to physical symptoms. All this will be done by gently encouraging them to consider these factors, and to engage in investigations to further reflect on discussions, this will lead to the development of a formulation.

Lewis (2013) asked cognitive behavioural therapists how they felt about working with the MUS group: the themes that arose were unfamiliarity, challenges in engagement and slow progress, although the clinicians did not necessarily consider the patients to be more difficult: part of the rationale for this book is to help with unfamiliarity and engagement. The core CBT skills needed across the board are completing a detailed assessment, measurement, collaboration, guided discovery and cognitive, behavioural and emotional change. With the MUS patients the additional skills are being able to work out the maintenance factors, when sometimes they may not be clear, being flexible around longer treatment duration and putting extra effort into relationship building. There are some protocols and treatment manuals that have been developed, but our experience is that it is most useful, in the MUS group, to work with the idiosyncratic maintenance factors. With the LTC population, CBT protocols for GAD, panic and depression can be slightly adjusted to allow for values-based goals, and for addressing 'realistic' NATs. There is a good evidence-based approach to health anxiety that can be used as a stand-alone treatment or integrated into other treatments.

## What is a suitable referral for CBT services, and what information is needed?

Patients may be sent to a CBT service by GPs, or allied health professionals in primary care such as physiotherapists and occupational therapists. From the physician group, neurologists, pain specialists and GI experts often refer, surgeons usually do not do. In our experience, the standard of referral is good: our colleagues do an excellent job in identifying psychological issues, and may try to work with the patients themselves, only referring on when this is challenging. It is also likely that there will be a lot of self-referrals to IAPT from this group, more likely in the LTC cohort. Sometimes particular medical colleagues have an interest in mental health, and refer a lot; other colleagues do not prioritise mental health, though they may have similarly needy patients. Mccrae, Correa, Chan, Jones and de Lusignan (2015) spoke to service leads in the IAPT pathfinder projects, where input was given to patients in these groups in various settings in England: most of the work was done by low-intensity therapists: psychological well-being and coping were targeted, it was felt that the participants benefitted, but the therapists needed further training with this less familiar group.

Because these patients may have existing medical problems, it is important that therapists have access to medical notes. On referral a patient may say something like 'doctors have told me I have a heart murmur', 'I'm breathless' and 'I have changes in my spine'; it is difficult to know from such descriptions whether the patient actually has a diagnosable medical condition. This medical information is important because we need to know whether the patient has been investigated and has had a medical reason for their symptoms excluded. Similarly, if we are asking the patient, for example, to exercise more, we need to be confident that there is no medical contraindication for this. It is therefore important that the psychological therapist understands the pre-existing medical condition, either from access to the notes or from discussion with the physician or GP. Ideally these patients should be referred with this medical summary, and a request from the GP as to what help they would like. One solution is for a letter to be written by the therapist asking the GP to summarise the patient's problems, and any relevant medical history. However, if none of this information is available, one would only go ahead if one were confident that the interaction of the psychological and physical symptoms was understood, and that MUS patients had been medically investigated.

It may be necessary, in order to encourage referrals and to help colleagues understand what we can offer, to provide formal presentations, publicity and informal discussions. Important educational points for our physical health colleagues are the difference between depression and normal sadness in long-term conditions, recognising health anxiety and referring it on, and the methods of engaging patients with MUS and where to refer them.

## Useful adaptations that can aid engagement

It is likely that we will need to make some adaptations in terms of assessing and indeed working with these patients who will be less likely to want to go to psychiatric clinics, so services should ideally be situated in GP practices, in IAPT buildings or in innovative settings like gyms. More attention than usual may need to be given to disabled access, parking or public transport availability, as this group will be less physically able. The use of SKYPE or video technology may be considered, especially for patients who struggle to physically travel to clinics, this is used more in the Covid situation and anecdotally has been found to be effective. Regarding the length of sessions, one might shorten the sessions, especially for patients who tire easily; however, we have typically done two-hour assessment sessions because we think that if patients have come a distance to see us then it is better to try and finish the assessment, and then work to engage them, as we might just have the one chance.

## Interpersonal engagement issues with MUS patients

When the patient comes to see the clinician, they may be keen, or not, in engaging with the service. The patients with MUS will think they are suffering from a medical illness, and will be surprised that no medical pathology has been found. When the suggestion is made by the GP or the physician or the therapist that psychological factors will be contributing to the symptoms, this news is likely to be treated with surprise in the first instance, and this may persist, and harden into disagreement, confusion or hostility. The engagement issues for the LTC and the MUS patients are different. The MUS patients may be happy to come to see you, but they may also be sceptical, hostile or anxious. These feelings are associated with thoughts like 'I don't understand how this (symptom) can be psychological, because it's so painful', 'If I see a psychologist I won't be taken seriously by the GP' and 'It's not fair that I've been forced to come here.' Our experience suggests that if the patient has got as far as coming to see the cognitive behavioural therapist, then the person beforehand has done an excellent job in engaging them, and they are likely to be willing to tell their story. Occasionally there is more explicit hostility to the assessment: we would suggest that in most cases it is better to just follow the normal CBT interview because this is an excellent way to engage the patient because of its comprehensive nature. Occasionally, it might be better to acknowledge the person's hostility, by asking 'how do you feel about being here today?'

The patient may be frustrated or hopeless that they have a set of distressing symptoms that no one has been able to explain. Houwen, Lucassen, Stappers, Assendelft and van Dulmen (2017) found that GPs and clinicians should pay empathic attention to the patient; treat him as an equal partner; and explore the symptoms of the MUS in depth. It is important to clarify the patient's understanding of why they have been referred, and what they hope to achieve from attendance. The clinician should make it clear that she does not think that the patient is 'mad' or that their symptoms are 'all in the mind', as these are commonly held and understandable fears of the patient (Kent & Mcmillan, 2009). In terms of patients with CFS, one study (Chew-Graham, Dowrick, Wearden, Richardson & Peters, 2010) found that patients were more likely to engage if one is 'ensuring that the patient feels accepted and believed, that they accept the diagnosis, and that the model implicated by the treatment offered to the patient matches the model of illness held by the patient'.

Another issue that could impede engagement is that because of the nature of MUS, the patient may have little actual understanding or awareness of psychological issues. The patient can present with few psychological stressors, an uneventful life history, and no clear psychological factors that can explain the symptoms. There could be a process of alexithymia here: this is an ancient Greek word that means not having the ability to recognise or describe one's emotions. The patient may have problems or issues that they are just not recognising, or down-play, or do not report. They are not consciously trying to conceal anything; they just have no awareness: this alexithymic trait has been associated with psychosomatic disorders (Charis & Panayiotou, 2018).

## The therapist worries they are missing a medical disorder in the MUS patient

It is also possible that a medical disorder has been missed or is emerging, and this is something that the patients and therapists can worry about, but it is reassuring to know that this is unlikely. An important study (Stone, Sharpe, Rothwell & Warlow, 2003) investigated this, following up patients with unexplained neurological conditions for a median of 12.5 years and found that only one of 60 patients had developed a neurological disorder. Another study (Skovenborg & Schröder, 2014) found that of 120 patients diagnosed with bodily distress syndrome (MUS), none of them had been misdiagnosed with actual serious medical disease after 3.2 years, although five patients had medical symptoms that had not been 'properly taken care of'. This means that it is unlikely that patients with MUS, or more specifically neurological MUS, have a serious underlying condition. If the cognitive behavioural therapist is concerned about certain symptoms (symptoms that are concerning are ones which are new, serious, disabling or have physical manifestations such as coughing up phlegm or bleeding), then it is reasonable to refer the patient back to the medical referrer for an opinion or discussion.

## Engagement issues with LTC and health anxiety patients

Generally building a therapeutic relationship with patients who have LTC is not too hard and a good introduction is: 'Thank you for coming today. I understand that you are suffering from some distressing symptoms/a named medical condition. I would like to make sense of this problem with you and how it is affecting you. I can see that these symptoms are disabling, we can hopefully help you cope with them better.' Relationship building is more challenging with patients who have health anxiety because in health anxiety the patient is often in two minds about attending: part of him worries about having an actual serious condition, so he is likely to be anxious about being seen in a mental health setting. His cognitions may be, 'If I come here, I won't be taken seriously by my GP', 'I want to prove this psychologist wrong, as it's risky to think of this as psychological' or 'maybe this person can reassure me about the symptom I'm currently worried about', the emotion of anxiety may be present. The person may seek reassurance or may give a 'doctored' account of their history, consciously, or less so. Another part of the patient may think 'these worries about my health are exaggerated, I need to seek psychological help', and they may engage in the interview more openly. Which attitude is met may depend on whether the patient has an active health worry when you speak to them. If the person settles in to the assessment interview that is fine, but if there is a sense that the person is holding back or seeking reassurance, one could say 'how do you feel about being here, what are your thoughts, how are they influencing your behaviour?'

## Encouraging family engagement

This is important in two ways: at assessment one can get information from the family that helps one understand the formulation. The benefit of additional information itself would be sufficient grounds for including the spouse, given how dependent the clinician is upon the narrative of the patient. And during treatment the relative may become a co-therapist, this being a person who aids the patient in doing their CBT programme. This involvement is particularly important in health anxiety, where the relative needs to understand the importance of not giving reassurance, whilst gently encouraging the patient to do their CBT homework. The relative can provide support and encouragement for the patient in doing their CBT homework, and discussion can be had about reducing overattentive relative behaviours if this is a problem (Woolfolk & Allen, 2007). A structure to do this is that every day the relative sits down with the patient and reviews the homework schedule, and encourages the patient to complete it.

## Controversies in MUS

Many patients believe that their symptoms are a genuine physical illness that is poorly understood by the medical establishment who in turn see these conditions as not easily explained by established disease processes, and therefore more likely to be psychological or bio-psychosocial. Social science literature has underlined the importance of patients seeking a valid diagnosis, at an experiential level, for legitimating illness, be it for legal, insurance and/or welfare purposes, or for the purpose of creating meaning. In particular, the social scientific literature has underlined how psychological explanations of symptoms can be a source of de-legitimation, as far as they are taken to imply that the illness is not as 'real' as physical disease (Greco, 2012). This can lead to conflicts between patients who are pursuing the disease model, and physicians who are discouraging this. This has led to activist groups, particularly CFS, strongly disagreeing with a CBT approach. For the typical cognitive behavioural therapist, it is not necessary to be fully understanding of the debates around MUS; it is more helpful to be aware of what the contributory factors are, how to recognise and measure them and how to consider whether they are relevant to the current problem. However, these issues are discussed further in Chapter 6.

## The use of supervision

The curriculum for the training with this group says that students should have a specialist supervisor, the authors also think this supervision should continue after initial training, and that supervision can follow the usual CBT approach. We would expect supervisors to be knowledgeable of and experienced in looking after these patients, and it will be helpful for the student to prepare a supervision question. Typical questions that are asked of us are: what is the formulation for this MUS patient, how much do you work at a problem or case level, how do you address the NATs in long-term conditions when they are so realistic, what goals do we negotiate here, what adaptations are made to treatment, and do we have to be more careful with exposure when patents have heart conditions? Most of these questions are addressed in the book.

## Chapter summary

One-third of the English population have a long-term condition, and a similar number of those have a mental health problem. The Covid epidemic could worsen this, but this is uncertain at the time of writing. Core CBT skills can be used in assessing and working with this group, and there is a desire to do this. The main patient groups are those with long-term conditions, medically unexplained symptoms and health anxiety. Therapists should ensure that practical adaptations are made, that therapist can access health records, and extra focus is put on engagement with the patient and family. CBT protocols can be used for depression and anxiety and long-term conditions, but idiosyncratic formulations are best with MUS.

# Chapter 2

# Assessment and formulation

The basic CBT assessment skills are used here. Once the therapeutic relationship has been established, the clinician will ask about the predisposing, precipitating and maintenance factors. The standard way to start is to ask for the 'main problem', and the patient may initially frame this as an emotional *or* a physical problem. Either way more time should be spent understanding the physical part of the cycle, which may be the trigger for emotional symptoms, or may be a consequence of emotional problems. It is important to listen carefully and empathically as patients describe their physical symptoms, moving on to ask for a specific instance of a time where they felt particularly anxious/depressed, or if they do not feel these emotions, then a time when the physical symptoms were particularly problematic.

## Special assessment focus if they have a medical problem

If the therapist knows that the person is suffering from a condition such as diabetes or cancer, it is more likely that they will be trying to understand why the person has struggled to adjust, has become depressed or has developed an anxiety disorder because of medical illness. With depression the therapist wants to understand themes of loss or failure, patterns of avoidance behaviour and negative automatic thoughts. With anxiety they would try to understand what the anxiety disorder is, and the maintenance factors. For example, if panic is suspected then catastrophic thinking, avoidance of situations that will trigger panic and safety behaviours used in situations needs to be understood; an example is the person with respiratory disease, who may have become panicky, triggered by breathlessness. In GAD, intolerance of uncertainty, positive beliefs about worry, problem avoidance and cognitive avoidance are the factors that need to be assessed, following the Dugas/Robichaud approach (Robichaud, Koerner & Dugas, 2019). For example, a person may have a diagnosis of cancer, and the GAD response may be worrying related to the uncertainty that this diagnosis brings, problems may be avoided, the person may believe that worry will help him cope with the cancer, and he may avoid potential distressing images of treatment or becoming more ill and the

DOI: 10.4324/9780367824433-4

person may feel out of control. Regarding PTSD, events like a cancer diagnosis, a spell in intensive care unit (ICU) or a life-changing accident can be a trigger for PTSD. With PTSD assessment will involve asking about negative thoughts about the accident and its aftermath, and patterns of avoidance, for example going back to the hospital or the accident site.

## Special assessment focus if the symptoms are medically unexplained

As mentioned previously the challenge here is to understand what maintenance factors are relevant, which is not always easy. This difficulty may be because alexithymia is blocking the person's awareness of these factors, or it may be the opposite problem in that the person seems to have a wide range of factors that could be implicated, but it is hard to decide which are the most relevant. We will now look at the standard CBT model of predisposing, precipitating and maintenance factors, as a way of structuring the assessment starting with the latter.

## Maintenance factors in MUS to look out for

There is considerable debate as to what these maintenance factors are, and it is fair to say that our understanding of this is incomplete. For the cognitive behavioural therapist it is important to be aware of the potential factors, and to try to assess these, and evaluate which ones it is most important to target. Deary, Chalder and Sharpe (2007) have supplied an excellent overview of these:

- *Sensitisation:* this means that there is a heightened physiological and behavioural response to aversive stimuli that has been previously met, often pain. This can be assessed by asking questions about the symptom: 'Have you experienced it before?', 'What was that experience like?' and 'Has that previous experience influenced how you now react to it now?'
- *Attentional processes*: there is increasing emphasis on this. Brown (2004) proposes a complex model that has a strong attentional element: unexplained symptoms arise when the chronic activation of stored representations in memory, called 'rogue representations', causes the attention system to select inappropriate information during attentional selection. These representations may be memories of earlier illness states, or illness in others. The symptomatic state is maintained by self-focused attention (amplifying the symptom); there is a misattribution of symptom to physical illness, an emotional change, worry and illness behaviour (Brown, 2004), so patients may become more aware and pre-occupied with, for example, their back pain. Rief, Hiller and Margraf (1998) suggest in their detailed study of cognition that patients may mistakenly believe symptoms to be important and pay attention to them, again amplifying them. The attentional state of the patient can be assessed as part of questioning about process, 'when you are aware of your symptoms

where does your attention go?', 'does that have any effect on the symptom?' Another way to think about this is to consider the concept of somatosensory amplification, elevated attention focusing is assumed to turn bodily sensations into symptoms and amplify the perception of mild somatic sensations and symptoms, creating a self-reinforcing circle (Barends et al., 2020)

- *Attribution:* the consensus as reported by Deary et al. (2007) is that attributions of vulnerability, lack of normalising and the symptoms representing a medical illness lead to increased symptom expression and illness behaviours. There is a surprising lack of research on specific thoughts, beliefs or personality factors in MUS. Rief et al. (1998) found that patients with health anxiety and somatisation had a self-concept of being weak and unable to tolerate stress, and had a style of catastrophising minor bodily complaints. Van Dijk et al. (2016), looking at the big five personality traits, suggests a specific personality profile for older somatising patients, with respect to 'neuroticism' that they have a higher level of neuroticism than controls, however, of interest, was the finding that the personality profile did not differ between older patients with medically unexplained and medically *explained* symptoms. So, the evidence is somewhat mixed as to whether thinking content/attribution is contributing to the MUS problems.

- *Behavioural responses:* aversive experiences will be avoided, so patients in pain will avoid the experience of pain and the triggering stimuli. This may be functional in acute pain, but in chronic pain the effect will be deconditioning and restricted lifestyle, which can contribute to depression (Vlaeyen & Linton, 2000). This state may be associated with thoughts such as, 'the pain will escalate unbearably', or will lead to damage. Patients with MUS will more generally restrict their lifestyle leading to more time spent on their own, increased rumination and lack of valued activities. Of course, the severity of the symptoms may make doing previously enjoyed activities harder. Assessment of all patient avoidant behaviours can be made by asking 'have you stopped doing things because of the symptoms; do you avoid things; why is that; help me understand?' Safety behaviours also need to be assessed, by asking more generally, 'what do you do to reduce the impact of the symptoms . . . what effect does this have on symptoms in the short and long term?' Examples of this in IBS are that the person, because of worries about being incontinent, may check where toilets are, restrict what he eats and drinks and spend excessive time on the toilet: these behaviours stop the person learning that the risks of incontinence are exaggerated, and by doing the behaviours he is giving himself a message that there is a real risk. Other behavioural responses that are met are 'overdoing it' behaviours. This means patients will drive themselves hard despite pain and fatigue. This can be a response to a sense that they must do activities when they have less pain or more energy, or it may also be influenced by rules such as 'If you don't do things perfectly, you're weak' or 'I mustn't be beaten': this 'overdoing it' behaviour may worsen symptoms. Patients with non-epileptic seizures, IBS, pain and fatigue are likely to be avoidant, because they feel that it will worsen their symptoms or put them in danger. Safety behaviour will be idiosyncratic to the symptoms and the beliefs, and the safety behaviours are problematic because they stop the person learning that their fears are exaggerated, and they also keep the person focused on the threat. Behavioural avoidance will lead to disuse and deconditioning and the person may withdraw not just from physical activity but may give up their role in life.

- *Sleep.* Although many of these patients complain about poor sleep (Morriss, Wearden & Battersby, 1997), there is little strong research evidence implicating this in MUS, so it is not clear whether this is a significant factor. Routine questions can be asked: 'what is your sleep like?', 'what time do you go to bed?', 'do you awake through the night?', 'what time do you get up?', 'is your sleep refreshing?' and 'is your sleep pattern associated with your problems?'. Some patients sleep excessively (especially with CFS), this could cause problems of deconditioning because of inactivity and time in bed.

- *Stressful events and experiences of abuse*: in our view, stressful events are a significant factor in most cases. There is a considerable literature on the effects of long-term stress in general, and in the MUS population, and we have observed many patients describing chronic stress and being anxious all the time. For example, there are increasing levels of stress, particularly in the months leading up to the onset of functional conditions, compared to depressed patients or controls (Nicholson et al., 2016). A systematic review of other functional disorders (including irritable bowel syndrome, chronic pelvic pain and somatisation disorder) also showed significantly increased rates of lifetime abuse in comparison to controls, and an association of abuse with symptom severity (Roelofs & Spinhoven, 2007). With chronic fatigue, more stressful events were found in the months preceding onset of CFS (Hatcher & House, 2003). However, research and clinical observation suggest that not all patients describe traumas and stress; this could be because of alexithymia and poor awareness in some cases. Emotional avoidance and/or suppression, particularly linked to anticipated emotional responses and unhelpful beliefs about those emotions, can be a maintenance factor, for the following reasons: there may be a lack of awareness of stressful events, so they are not dealt with these effectively and they become chronic, or the emotions associated with them are not processed. So, the patient may say or think 'I suffer from headaches' and not acknowledge that he is suffering significant stress. This alexithymia may be driven by personality traits or beliefs such as 'if I don't do things perfectly, there's no point in doing it', 'showing emotions is a sign of weakness' or 'Don't burden people with problems' or 'I'm not the kind of person who gets stressed.' At assessment, the therapist needs to explore the life events the person has experienced, how he has dealt with these, whether he expresses and acknowledges his feelings and any link with the presenting problem. Questionnaires like the Toronto alexithymia scale may help this (Bagby, Parker & Taylor, 1994).

- *How stress effects the individual:* the literature on the effects of chronic stress on the body is helpful here: Homoeostasis is the idea that the body has an ideal level of oxygen, an ideal degree of acidity, ideal temperature and so on and the brain will regulate physiological variables in response to, or in anticipation of a threat (Sapolsky, 2004) by the secretion of hormones, or the activation of certain parts of the nervous system. A *stressor* is anything in the outside world that knocks one out of homoeostatic/allostatic balance, and the stress response is what the body does to re-establish homoeostasis. For evolutionary reasons, the body's stress response is more ideally suited to the zebra or lion; it is short-sighted, inefficient and urgent: blood pressure will rise and the immune system will be suppressed, there will be more energy used than stored and the person will fatigue more easily (Sapolsky, 2004). It may be that when the physiological stress response is turned on, it becomes difficult to turn off again, and has general wear-and-tear effects on various physiological systems (Sapolsky, 2004). McEwen (1998) also discusses this concept stating the most common allostatic responses involve the sympathetic nervous systems and the HPA axis. *The HPA axis* (hypothalamus pituitary adrenal) is part of the body's response to stress: the HPA axis alters energy metabolism, influences immune functioning and affects both energy and mood. There may be a problem with prolonged activation of this response. Cleare (2004) has looked at HPA thoroughly in CFS, and found no actual dysfunction, but possible subtle effects.
- *Emotion:* There is a strong association between what is often called high negative affect (excessive anxiety and depression) and MUS (Constantinou, 2018). However, we also need to consider the emotional response in long-term conditions which is usually that of depression, sometimes guilt. So, in assessment of long-term conditions, we are assessing whether the emotional response would meet the diagnostic criteria for depression, in essence that it is excessive and prolonged.
- *Medication and substance misuse*: our observation is that patients do not always use medications well, or less commonly they may be taking illegal substances that are contributing to the symptoms, and this needs to be assessed. For example, opioid-like medications are used in pain, but there has been recent realisation of the problems they may cause in chronic pain. There is a guideline from the United States that recommends that opioid equivalents are not the first choice of medications for non-malignant chronic pain, and if they are used, clinicians should consider treatment goals, minimal dosing and how to stop them if they are ineffective (Dowell, Haegerich & Chou, 2016). When assessing patients, one should always ask about their use of prescribed medication, also about use of illicit substances, and in doing so, one should also remember that it is now easier for patients to access medication over the internet without prescription. With opioids the problems are excessive drowsiness (that may restrict the person living a full life), the risk of overdose and the habituation effect with increased dosages needed for effect.

Sometimes medications are not taken in a very logical way: for example, analgesics should be taken regularly to reduce the risks of pain building up rather than as required, and sometimes patients seem to be taking the medications at the wrong time of the day, or medications have not been reviewed for a long time. It is appreciated that not all cognitive behavioural therapists have the expertise to review these drugs, but in this field, it is important to have a working knowledge of typical drugs that are prescribed, and a sense whether they used appropriately or rationally. Sometimes the clinician meets the very stoic patient whom they feel would receive help from a medication regime, but they resist this because they think, 'I'll get addicted . . . I'm not the kind of person to take drugs . . . I won't be able to tolerate the side-effects.' These attitudes can potentially be explored by the therapist.

- *Secondary gain/fear of recovery*: most therapists working with these patients agree that sometimes there is a secondary gain for having the symptoms. This means that not having to go to an unwanted job; receiving benefits; attention from family; insurance or litigation payments are potential rewards for having the symptoms. Operant conditioning would explain that the reward of, say, receiving the benefits encourages the illness behaviours, and occasionally patients deliberately exaggerate the symptoms, but most of the time this process seems out of awareness. Sharpe et al. (2010) showed that in unexplained neurological symptoms at one year receiving disability benefits was a factor that predicted poor outcome (alongside expectation of non-recovery and non-attribution of symptoms to non-psychological factors). Some of the factors that would indicate secondary gain are: the symptoms do not seem as severe as the patient says; there is a very attentive spouse or family; a history of dependent traits; financial benefits that would make getting well very disadvantageous; strong pressure for the therapist to write reports or provide statements for benefits, insurance or legal agencies; the patient's story is confused, inconsistent or hard to understand. One must tread carefully at the assessment stage, as this line of questioning can alienate the patient such that they do not come back. It's best to explore this delicately when the therapeutic relationship is stronger, and questions that could be asked are, 'Do you have any fears of getting better . . . do you feel stuck with your symptoms . . . have you heard of the sick role, do you think this idea relates to you . . . I could understand if you were fearful of going back to work, is this the case with you at all?' (see the final chapter).

## Precipitating factors in MUS

There is an overlap here with the maintenance section discussion of stressful events. Steinbrecher and Hiller (2011) found a higher number of life events were a predictor of MUS in primary care. Organic illness and stressful work conditions have also been described by Henningsen, Zipfel, Sattel and Creed (2018). As part of the CBT assessment, it is routine to ask about predisposing factors, by asking 'tell me about when the problem started . . . what was going on in your life . . . did you have any stressful events (including work), or physical health problems . . . do you think these factors are relevant to your current problems?' Bonvanie, Janssens, Rosmalen and Oldehinkel (2017) found a clear link between stressful life events and MUS in adolescents.

## Predisposing factors in MUS

MUS are associated with being female, younger and self-employed, and they are more common in lower social and economic backgrounds. They are correlated with past and current episodes of anxiety and depression (Nimnuan, Hotopf & Wessely, 2001). The paper by Roelofs and Spinhoven (2007) evaluates evidence concerning the relationship between MUS and trauma, showing that trauma in the form of childhood sexual, physical and/or emotional abuse is particularly common in patients with MUS, although it is not universally found. Early traumatisation may serve as a *predisposing* factor. This factor makes the central stress system more vulnerable to the effects of later stressors that, in turn, may serve as precipitating factors for symptom onset, and affect symptom manifestation (McEwen, 1998).

## Cultural factors in MUS

Simon, Gater, Kisely and Piccinelli (1996) showed that unexplained somatic symptoms (most often aches and pains) are consistently common in a range of cultures, and across cultures are associated with anxiety and depression, anxiety slightly more so. The specific manifestation of these symptoms and the labelling of them will vary. Whilst being sensitive to cultural factors, we suggest that assessment and treatment are essentially the same across cultures.

## A suggested structure for assessment

- Introduce self and the purpose of the assessment. Refer to the earlier notes and the referral letter.
- Ask about the main problem if the patient describes physical symptoms, and then get some details of these. One can check at this point if the person is suffering from an illness like COPD or diabetes. If the person describes psychological symptoms such as anxiety, get some details of these.
- Ask for an example of when the symptoms were most problematic. If they describe anxiety/depression, ask what the triggering event was (it may be a physical symptom or a general stressor); ask them what cognitions they had when they experienced that symptom, inference chain this to the 'hot thought', then broaden this out to other processes such as attention, image/memory, worry/rumination and thinking errors. Then ask about behavioural responses including what they avoided, what they did in the situation to keep

them safe, reassurance seeking behaviours and escape behaviours. If their example starts with physical symptoms, then one wants to know if there was an emotional response, then the other parts of the vicious circle are assessed as described.

- Ask them about all triggers for the symptoms.
- Ask what they would like to be different, what their goals are.
- Ask what the onset of the problem was and how the problem has changed over the years.
- One then wants to know about what are called modifiers: medication use (including when medication was last reviewed, whether the medication is helpful); alcohol use in weekly units; taking of illegal drugs; smoking tobacco; what they eat; and use of caffeine.
- Next, ask about their personal life history thinking about precipitating factors.
- Our practice is to be structured asking about: 'what is your previous medical history?', 'what is your previous psychiatric history?' and 'do you have any involvement with the police or the legal system?'
- Then, 'tell me about your living arrangements?', 'do you have any financial problems?' and 'what are your hobbies and interests?'
- Followed by 'tell me about your mother and father, their ages, mental and psychiatric history and your relationship with them. Likewise, your siblings'.
- We would say: 'did you have any problems at your birth, and reaching your milestones?' 'What was the family atmosphere like as a child. Were there experiences of illness in the family? How did you and your family react to those?'
- 'What secondary school did you go to, did you experience bullying, truancy or absences?' 'Did you get your qualifications?'
- 'What did you do when you left school? What is your employment history? Are you working now? Tell me about your job.'
- 'What serious relationships have you had? Are you with someone now? How is that relationship? How does she/he react to your problems?'
- 'Do you have children? Tell me a bit about them.'
- 'What is your sex life like, have you experienced sexual abuse?'
- 'Are you religious or spiritual?'
- 'What is your personality like? How do you see yourself and the world? How do you get on with people?'
- We would conclude with a mini-mental state exam: our observations of their posture, speech and manner. We would ask about features of depression (and suicidal thoughts), the anxiety disorders (particularly health anxiety, PTSD, trauma and GAD), any body image problems, any abnormal eating and any features of psychosis. How much we went in to these topics here would depend in the patient's answer and whether we had gone into this earlier.

This is a time-consuming assessment, but the authors believe these questions will help us most to understand the problem and help the patient feel that we are working hard to fully appreciate how tough it is. At a basic level we are trying to understand the predisposing, precipitating and maintenance factors.

So, when asking about the maintenance factors we (the assessors) are think-ing about the following: 'what is the relationship between the triggering factors and the patient symptoms?' An obvious one would be a simple 'every time I feel stressed, I get a headache', but that relationship is rarely that simple. We would at least be looking out for history of stressful events, that have some interacting relationship with the symptoms. We would be trying to work out if the patient was engaging in behaviours such as avoidance, safety behaviours, abnormal postures and physical guarding that could be contributing to the problem. We would want to understand whether the patient would meet the diagnostic criteria for a mental health disorder such as depression, PTSD or panic.

## How to formulate MUS patients

The first thing is to establish whether the patients have any of the maintenance fac-tors described earlier. When this is done, the task is to see if these factors are likely

*Table 2.1* Common formulation problems and actions

| Common formulation problems | Actions |
| --- | --- |
| The patient does not present psychological factors | There are two possibilities here. One is that psychological factors are not relevant to the presentation. The other is that the person is not very aware of the factors or is downplaying them because of poor emotional awareness. One can try to assess for alexithymia, questions could be 'Are you in touch with your emotions . . . can you express your feelings . . . if you were sad could you say . . . are you emotionally aware?', the therapist can give the patient a diary to see if further links can be made. Speaking to the family about whether they think there are links can be useful. The Toronto alexithymia scale may be used here. |
| The patient does present psychological factors, but it is not clear whether they are relevant to the problem | We would look out for timeline links. This may be that the maintenance factors are present around the time the patient has the symptoms. This may be broad (my IBS was a bit worse when I had that period of stress), or more acute (when I focused on the pain yesterday it was worse). However, sometimes the patient says, 'I was coping quite well, but when the stress became easier, the symptoms started': this is a manifestation of pushing on and coping, ignoring the symptoms or pushing through them at the time. Again, a diary may help. |

| Common formulation problems | Actions |
|---|---|
| The patient presents many psychological factors, but it is not clear which ones are relevant | A collaborative approach will be most helpful here. We would also be tempted to think that if there are a lot of psychological issues then it is likely that some of these will be contributing to the MUS presentation. The therapist just needs to use his clinical skills to try to judge what seems most relevant, and often time is needed to allow things to become clearer. Sometimes the therapist needs to be tolerant of uncertainty in that a comprehensive formulation is not very present, but there are clearly issues that the patient wants to work on. |

to be causing or contributing to the presenting problem (e.g. problems like IBS, non-epileptic seizures and chronic pain). This process can range from straight forward to quite challenging. A collaborative approach is helpful as always, a good question would be 'do you think this is likely to be a factor in your problems'. If one gets a lot of initial agreement, then it becomes clear what factors should be worked on. Issues of MUS are discussed further in Chapter 7.

## Assessing suitability and engaging patient with the formulation

As usual with CBT there are some things that make the patient 'suitable', that should be considered: they have some awareness of their own thoughts and feelings; they want to work on a current problem; they accept the need to do homework between sessions; and there is some confidence in the formulation as a reasonable description of the predisposing, precipitating and maintenance factors.

Sometimes the clinician can be more confident in their formulation, but the patient is more sceptical; this will be more common in MUS/HA. Obviously, the therapist would explore this collaboratively, trying to understand the patient's concerns and this is more likely to be around the patient struggling to see that psychological factors can be at play when the symptoms are so strong and disabling.

What can be done to help engage the patient with the CBT formulation: one could use a simple example and try to apply it to the person's more complex presentation. For example, we could say 'Have you ever had a tension headache?' That is an example of stress factors influencing a physical process. It is also possible to explain symptoms at different levels: there is a *physiological* process likely to be muscle contraction in the head and neck; one could also see it at the level of there being several *stressful events* that influence physiological processes; we can also consider the *behavioural response* such as dealing with the stressor, or ignoring it, or taking analgesics, and avoiding the triggers, and we can think how the behavioural response would influence the symptom. We could use the computer metaphor: 'with these symptoms that you've got, it may be helpful to think about the computer. There is nothing wrong with the hardware, but there is with the software, so we need to understand what's wrong there and try to fix it. What's your view?' Occasionally you may get no agreement on the formulation; it is possible to say to the patient to try CBT and see if it helps. If the patient does not agree with the formulation or trying treatment, then it may be worth leaving the door open for them a future date.

As said earlier, it is harder to do formulations with the MUS group, and you or the patient or both may have varying amounts of confidence in your formulation. It is possible to continue with treatment if both of you feel that the formulation is reasonably accurate, even though you might not be 100% sure. It may be that material appears that helps fine tune your first hypothesis. With the LTC and health anxiety group the formulation will be easier, so a modified version of the standard protocols (Depression/PTSD/GAD, etc.) can usually be used.

## MUS formulation example

Here is an extract from my (PK) letter to referrer: 'Thank you for referring this patient, Margaret, who presents with quite complex problems. The primary problem was jumpy, restless legs, which are there constantly, including through the night. There does not appear to be any trigger for this problem: her legs start stamping up and down, going faster and faster, and this movement jars and causes her considerable pain. To relieve this, she paces up and down, which helps a bit, and sometimes walks very slowly, which also seems to help. This problem occurs constantly, with few breaks. She has tried to manage it by holding her legs still but cannot consistently do so. She describes her emotional state as being alright, and not too stressed currently, but she is anxious about the pain that she gets.

She presented to me as quite agitated. She did not look very well. She was pacing up and down. She presented her history quite well. She denied feeling depressed; she said she does have suicidal thoughts but would not act on them. The problem with her legs has got significantly worse since she had an operation 6 months ago. Before that she says she was functioning a lot better and was driving, which she cannot do now. She tends to stay at home, and sometimes does not even get dressed. She feels that her mood is lower because of the effect of pain, and her inability to live a normal life. The impact is also that she gets little sleep because she will find herself kicking her husband in the bed, so she does not actually go to bed. The other impact is that the problem has got so bad that her children have had to press down on her legs to restrain them. She also suffers from considerable physical problems. She has a chronic lung condition, she has had two MIs in the past, and mild arthritis. She is on several medications as described in her GP's letter, including medications to control her legs. She feels that taking dihydrocodeine and diazepam does help temporarily. She smokes 20 cigarettes a day. She drinks 10 cups of coffee a day. She does not drink alcohol.

The onset of the problem was 9–10 years ago, she had very mild jumpy legs, which came unexpectedly, but this problem was not a major issue for her. However, 6 months ago after she had an operation, she describes a significant deterioration in her symptoms. In between these dates she has had two tragic bereavements of her older children on separate occasions. The second time she told me this story, when I saw her again, she was quite emotional describing her loss. Her goals for therapy are to get rid of her symptoms.'

This is an unusual presenting problem. A first consideration is whether it could be a medical problem, as there is such a thing as restless legs syndrome, but conversations with medical colleagues indicated they did not think it was medical. She is suffering major long-term conditions but was not particularly struggling with these. The main problem was the restless legs: it is possible that these are manifestations of anxiety, the course of adrenaline and cortisone in her system with flight response making her want to move/run. She paces up and down in response to this, which reduces the distress but may maintain the problem through the process of negative re-enforcement. The patient says she feels worse when she does not do it but it may be that trying to stop it in the longer term is the right thing to do. Also, the patient does not describe a lot of current anxiety, but on observations seems anxious and she has a lot of serious medical problems to contend with. Possible alexithymia here?

What about the tragic bereavements? This would seem a factor, but the timeline does not match. She also feels that she has dealt as well as she can with this through counselling at the time. The patient's perspective is that she is struck by how this problem got a lot worse after her operation. This is difficult to make sense of from a medical perspective, and she did not find the operation particularly challenging. Ultimately, we felt we could move forward on some further CBT grief counselling as this was likely to be a factor. My colleague has taken this forward, and the restless legs symptoms seem the same the patient is emotionally benefitting from the approach.

Step-by-step issues in case formulation: Kuyken, Padesky and Dudley (2008) usefully divide the process of case formulation into descriptive, cross-sectional and longitudinal. Descriptive means relatively simple descriptions of the presenting problem in terms of associations or dynamic interactions. A commonly used descriptive approach would be Padesky's five areas approach (Padesky, 2020), describing the interaction of the triggers, cognition, emotion, physiology and behaviour. Next level is cross-sectional which includes triggers and factors that maintain the problem across situations, and the final area is longitudinal, which brings in early experiences, developmental history (including of illness), core beliefs and rules for living.

## Formulation Procedure:

- Decide a list of all *current problems* and outline these in cognitive behavioural terms (*Description*).

- Take each presenting problem and make sense of it with the patient in terms of the links between triggers, cognition, emotion, physiology and behaviour (*cross-sectional*).
- Link presenting problems to case factors such as early experiences, or core beliefs and rules for living, early trauma and so on (*longitudinal*).

## Formulation tips when there is MUS:

- Think about the way that emotion can drive symptoms.
- Think about the way the person may be unaware of, or deny psychological states (but be open minded as to whether this is happening).
- Consider how avoidant, and safety, and poor coping behaviours are worsening the symptoms.
- If the therapist is not sure whether there is a psychological issue: do lots of questionnaires; speak to GP and family; get the patient to keep a diary. If you discharge them keep an open door.
- Accept your own uncertainty that when you develop a formulation with MUS, this will be more tentative than usual.

*Table 2.2* Common presentations and maintenance factors, as seen in clinical practice or in the literature

| Common presentations | Common maintenance factors |
|---|---|
| Chronic fatigue syndrome | Stress; boom and bust; perfectionism; avoidance/deconditioning. |
| Chronic pain | Avoidance/deconditioning: medication misuse; fear and catastrophising. |
| Non-epileptic seizures | Response to trauma, pain and stress; dissociation/freezing; excessive avoidance of triggers; causes sometimes unclear. |
| Irritable bowel syndrome | Stress; fear of incontinence; shame about symptoms. |
| Voice problems | Effects of stress on the voice; abuse/trauma with fear of speaking up leading to aphonia. |
| Conversion disorders, also known as functional neurological disorders (where there are problems with sensory or motor function) | Stress; trauma; disuse and abnormal use of part of the body that is affected; secondary gain. |
| Skin conditions | Stress. |
| Factitious disorder | Patterns of behaviour of seeking medical attention and achieving safety and control through this; difficult early experiences in the medical and other domains; personality factors. |

## LTC formulation examples

Example 1 Jim: list of established *current problems*: Jim is a 57-year-old man with a history of a panic disorder. Over the last year he has developed COPD, with cough, breathlessness on exertion and tiredness. He has been sent to CBT because he has been becoming increasingly anxious about his symptoms, but his GP says his COPD is stable. When his symptoms flare up, he gets panicky about them, his cognitions are 'my breathing's terrible, I could stop breathing, this is horrible, I will suffocate and die', he feels very anxious which produces dizziness, breathlessness and racing heart. His behaviour is to stay at home and avoid activity, to take inhalers more than is necessary and to want his wife to stay with him, and he checks his pulse and counts his breaths. His attention is on his breathing all the time, and he has memories of when he had panic attacks before, which was horrible.

*Cross-sectional formulation*: this case is not too difficult to formulate: the therapist would quickly see that negative thoughts such as 'I will suffocate and die', will be triggered by his COPD symptoms, which will then worsen his anxiety, and potentially worsen the breathlessness symptoms, memories of his first attack could also worsen his anxiety here. The safety behaviours and avoidance are stopping him learning that the feared consequence is unlikely to occur, and making him over-preoccupied with his symptoms, at the expense of engagement in his life. A Padesky five-area formulation could be presented here emphasising these links. A full *case formulation* is not needed here, as the information gathered does not suggest that core beliefs and rules for living are relevant to our understanding.

A treatment plan based on psycho-education about panic was developed, and the consideration of cautious exposure targets was discussed.

Example 2 Fiona: current problems: she describes being exhausted, and feeling ill all the time. She has joint pains and headaches. It is worse if she does things. She has blood pressure problems, going in spikes, and she has been told she has hypertension. She is quite worried about hypertension and that she could have a stroke. Fiona is not sure what the cause of the symptoms is, she does feel that there is something wrong and she is anxious about this. She not only engages in some health anxiety-related behaviours such as checking and watching her symptoms, but also tries to use her previously learned CBT techniques. She is a little bit avoidant in doing things, mainly because of fatigue, but also tries to push herself by taking walks.

The onset of the problem was 2016. She had a hearing problem, which doctors did not initially diagnose; she was then given a serious diagnosis for this, this has damaged her trust in doctors. She has had fatigue for a year and hypertension for three years. In terms of her goals, she wants help to get things in perspective, deal with anxiety, to do more, be less prickly, not to worry in general – she worries about a wider range of things than just health anxiety. She has an alcohol consumption of 60 units week. She has quite negative views about herself, for example she will say, 'I'm an awful person, I'm selfish.'

This is a more complex presentation: the problem list could be said to be, exhaustion, aches and pains, health anxiety, hypertension, excessive alcohol consumption. At the level of the *cross-sectional formulation*, we need to try and work out how problems interact, and do this collaboratively. Regarding the fatigue and aches and pains a maintenance factor is chronic anxiety, the patient thought this was a possibility, but was not sure. It is possible that avoidance of activity and a boom-and-bust pattern could be worsening the fatigue. The health anxiety tended to be triggered by pain and episodes of hypertension, and made worse by catastrophic thinking and safety behaviours. The hypertension was a medical problem, but we thought there could be a link to chronic stress. That was a background process of worry that was making the anxiety worse. Alcohol consumption was excessive, impairing her ability to live a normal life and potentially damaging health in other ways. At the level of longitudinal formulation their work or beliefs such as 'I'm an awful person', and 'I don't trust the medical profession', the latter leading to a lack of trust in the medical system which could impinge on the therapeutic relationship with professionals and damage trust further.

Example 3 Robert: he describes having a dystonic movement disorder; he has been to neurology about this and had an MRI scan. He has been told that it is a 'software' rather than a 'hardware' issue. He has abnormal movements, particularly on the right side of his body, the right side of his face drops, his head goes over to the side, he twists his hand and feet and the right side can twist as well. He has a strange sensation – he can feel hypersensitive in his limbs. These symptoms occur 3–4 times a week and last from hours to days, the longest he has had without an attack is 7 days, but the pattern can vary in intensity and frequency. He has struggled to pin down specific triggers, but does think there is a relationship with stress and also perfectionism. He describes a history of generalised anxiety disorder and has had two rounds of CBT in primary care, which has been helpful, and worked on perfectionism and stress control. A typical episode was the weekend before: he got up went shopping with his wife, then felt strange in his right side, so he lay down on the sofa but it got worse and his hand and foot hurt. He took diazepam and waited for it to kick in, this eventually relaxed his muscles but also put his to sleep, and it only works for a brief period. He got up the next morning and his limbs were painful and cramping, he tries to do his activities and ignore it, but sometimes this is difficult and he will have to stop doing things, this is a prediction that he will not be able to do them. The impact of the problem is that he is taking time off work, he has quite an elevated level of pain, and he has also had to cancel private engagements, mostly because of embarrassment. This is more of problem if people do not know, and less so if people do know about the condition. He has cognitions such as, 'what are they thinking about now?' and 'I look weird.' He describes being anxious over the last decade, he feels he is not living up to what he could be, he should do things better, and feels a bit of a failure, letting people down. Because of perfectionism and worry, he will tend to avoid challenges, such as meetings, doing reports, small DIY jobs. The onset of the movement problem was 4½ years ago, he had changed jobs just beforehand his face suddenly fell, he got a fright thinking it might be a stroke and went to ED. It happened again sometime later. The right side of his body got worse, more often. He struggled to find strategies to deal with this. He does try to exercise but has reduced this compared to his earlier level of fitness. His goals are not to have the movements.

We agreed a problem list, the main one being that this dystonic movements: through research and then conversation, we established that this was a movement disorder in which muscles contacted uncontrollably, that can have various causes from brain damage or degeneration to psychological factors, in his case he had accepted from the neurologists that the brain was healthy. A second problem was anxiety, both generalised and social. There is a probable link between anxiety, and a worsening of the dystonia and this worsened the social anxiety. We collaboratively created a generic five areas formulation. Triggering events was stressful events particularly at work, this tends to make the dystonic movements worse. The movements caused pain (physiology), and made him more self-conscious (cognitive process). His (behavioural) response was to take time off work and to avoid, which may or may not have been helpful. His thinking style wise to worry about situations. He often worked long hours in quite a perfectionist way (behaviour). He engaged in negative automatic thoughts (cognition), such as 'I'm weird' and 'what are they thinking about me'. At a basic level we were able to agree how these factors could interact, and as we continue therapy, we teased out the nuances of this and then a (case) formulation was developed looking at issues of self-esteem, having a chronic movement problem, having a history of anxiety, and having some problematic core beliefs and rules.

## Does the clinician need to pay special attention to suicide risk?

In Druss and Pincus (2000), 5.5% of American respondents had made a suicide attempt (self-harm), 8.9% of those with a general medical illness, and 16.2% of those with 2 or more medical conditions had attempted suicide. In models controlling for major depression, depressive symptoms, alcohol use, and demographic characteristics, presence of a general medical condition predicted 1.3 times increase in likelihood of suicidal ideation; more specifically, pulmonary diseases (asthma, bronchitis) were associated with a two-thirds increase in the odds of lifetime suicidal ideation. Cancer and asthma were each associated with a more than 4-fold increase in the likelihood of a suicide attempt. With completed suicide, increased risk was seen for HIV/AIDS, malignant neoplasms as a group, head and neck cancers, Huntington disease, multiple sclerosis, peptic ulcer, renal disease, spinal cord injury, and systemic lupus erythematosus. Being a burden was the key variable in increasing suicide risk in chronic pain patients (Kanzler, Bryan, McGeary & Morrow, 2012). Suicide risk is higher if they have a medical condition at a younger age (Scott et al., 2010). In older age general suicide risk increases, and although physical illness and functional impairment increased risk, this seems to be mediated by depressive disorder (Conwell, Duberstein & Caine, 2002). Suicide risk should always be assessed.

## Chapter summary

The relevant maintenance factors in this MUS group are sensitisation, stress and HPA axis dysfunction, attentional processes, attribution problems, behavioural responses, sleep issues, emotional factors, medication and substance abuse and fear of recovery: these need to be identified and addressed in treatment.

# Chapter 3

# Measuring problems, establishing suitability and negotiating goals

So, although we are focusing on CBT in this book, it is important to firstly look at whether CBT would be most effective for the person's presenting problem or possible other therapies would be better or low intensity would be better. We will discuss the low-intensity approach in detail in the next chapter.

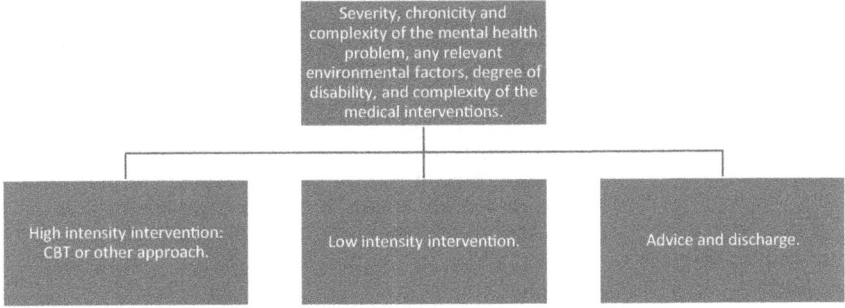

*Figure 3.1* Pathway after assessment

After we have done the assessment described in Chapter 1, and we have developed a collaborative formulation we have now got to the position of taking the person into treatment. The next thing to do will be questionnaires. These should be both idiographic, where the person keeps a record of their problems, and standard questionnaires, such as the GAD-7 and the PHQ-15 When considering questionnaires, it is often useful to think about more general questionnaires which may be administered routinely in that service, and questionnaires that measure the severity of the presenting problem.

Here is a table of some of the most used ones.

DOI: 10.4324/9780367824433-5

*Table 3.1* Questionnaires

| Presenting problem | Questionnaire | Notes |
|---|---|---|
| Depression | PHQ-9 | A standard IAPT measure for mild, moderate, and severe depression. |
| Anxiety | GAD-7 (Spitzer, Kroenke, Williams & Löwe, 2006) | A standard IAPT measure for anxiety |
| MUS | PHQ-15(Kroenke & Spitzer, 2002) | The PHQ-15 is a brief, self-administered questionnaire that may be useful in screening for somatisation and in monitoring somatic symptom severity in clinical practice and research. |
| Fatigue | Chalder fatigue scale (Chalder et al., 1993) | A standard measure of fatigue |
| IBS | Francis IBS scale (Francis, Morris & Whorwell, 1997) | A standard measure of IBS |
| Across disorders impact of the problem | Work and social adjustment scale (Mundt, Marks, Shear & Greist, 2002) | Measures impact on life and functioning |
| Pain | PAIN visual analogue scale (Carlsson, 1983) | Simple measure of pain |
| Pain | Short form McGill (Dworkin et al., 2009) | Rates aspects of pain on 1–3 severity scale. |
| Long-term conditions general | Long-term conditions scale | Scale in development |
| Cardiac conditions | Nothing currently available | |
| Non epileptic seizures | Nothing currently available | |
| COPD | Nothing currently available | |
| Health anxiety/ hypochondriasis/ illness anxiety disorder | Health Anxiety inventory (Abramowitz, Deacon & Valentiner, 2007) | Measurement of health anxiety |

There are several ways that this information can be used, for example it can aid a diagnosis in some cases. So, if the patient had a positive score on the PHQ (cut off over 10) it would support a conclusion of depression. Consideration must be given to the fact that this group will have physical symptoms so certain symptoms that are associated with anxiety (raised heart rate) may be a symptom of a medical problem, and vice versa. So, one needs to be a little cautious when analysing questionnaire data in this group. The other advantage of this data is that it allows the clinician to monitor changes in the presenting problem.

Another source of information is to ask the patient to complete a questionnaire that tracks the frequency of their symptoms/problems: the rationale for this is to help the patients and therapist to understand the contextual factors that are influencing this. When one is thinking about this one has the choice to use idiographic diaries that have been used for each disorder or to use a more generic diary. Here is an example of a generic diary.

*Table 3.2* Generic diary

| Date/Time: | Describe the symptoms | What were the factors: stress, thinking, emotional, medical, that influenced the symptoms? | How did you respond behaviourally to the symptoms? |
|---|---|---|---|
|  |  |  |  |
|  |  |  |  |
|  |  |  |  |

One would say to the patient: 'I would like you to fill in this diary for two weeks in order that we both get a better picture of the factors that are influencing your symptoms. Every time you get a symptom please fill in the diary at the time. Are you able to do that? Will there be any problems doing this? Shall we do an example in the session now?' Typically, patients will be willing to do this.

If one is treating anxiety or depression in an LTC then it is better getting hold of the specific diaries that are included in the protocols. When the diaries are returned there is a skill in extracting the information. A good collaborative question is 'What did you learn from doing the diary', and in the diary as given in Table 3.2 you can try to see whether external factors such as stress, health problems, relationship issues are the precursors of the symptom. Sometimes this is obvious, other times it is harder to see a pattern.

Typical things to look out for as triggers are: a period of stress; relationship issues; work issues; 'benefits' issues; physical illness; viruses. Likewise, one can begin to see whether the person's behaviour is helpful or contributing to the problem, as described in the following table:

*Table 3.3* Behavioural responses

| Unhelpful behaviour/response | Helpful behaviour/response |
|---|---|
| Avoidance. | Facing the situation and dealing with it. |
| Excessive help seeking. | Fostering independence but accepting help if required. |
| Reassurance seeking. | Accepting good advice when it has been given. |
| Safety seeking behaviours. | Not seeking safety when there is no danger. |
| Avoidant of exercise; obsessive exercise for unhealthy reasons. | Healthy exercise. |
| Eating unhealthily, weight obsessed, overeating. | Eating well |
| Denying the reality of the condition, engaging with quack medicine, using all resources looking for explanation or cure. | Accepting the reality of the condition you have whilst trying to maximise your health. |
| Avoiding going to the Doctors, or going excessively. | Going to medical appointments and accepting reasonable guidance. |

If it may be worth continuing the diary as two weeks may not be long enough to see patterns. One would collaborate with the patient as to whether this is worthwhile. The next stage in the process in completing the Problem and Goals sheet. We do this collaboratively with the patient before any treatment is provided. The rationale for this is to help the patient describe and list the problems that they want to work on, and then to agree SMART (Specific, measurable, achievable, realistic, time limited) goals. The problems are then measured in terms of the impact they are having on the person's life, and the goals are measured in terms of how much the person has achieved the goal in percentage terms.

With health anxiety it is not usually too difficult to develop a problem statement, for example: 'When I get an unusual symptom, I tend to worry it is the first sign of cancer, this makes me more anxious, I feel breathless and dizzy which fuels my worries about cancer. I respond to this by checking my pulse and breathing, many times a day, and I go to the GP excessively for reassurance about my symptoms.' Appropriate goals here would be: 'I will appraise new symptoms realistically; I will only go to the GP if I have symptoms which I consider new, severe or persistent, or a combination of these; I will only go to the GP if I think they would want to see me. I will not seek re-assurance if I am excessively worried about my health; I will not take, my pulse, scan my body, count my breathing (etc) for the purposes of reassurance.'

With long-term conditions a problem statement could be: 'I suffer from Parkinson's disease, my mood has lowered in response to this associated with thoughts, "I can't live my life, I won't get better so nothing is worth it, I can't live like this." My behavioural response is to avoid valued activities, and to spend excessive time in bed which can worsen my mood further.' Possible goals here are: 'I will work out which elements of my thoughts are distorted, and I will challenge these; If my thoughts are realistic, I will work out how I can live a valuable and enjoyable life around my health problems; I will seek the appropriate level of help from other people, and accept it when it is offered; I will engage in activity scheduling to maximise the activities that are valuable, masterful and pleasurable; I will get the best care from the health care system; I will face the fact that my own life will come to an end and discuss my feelings about this.'

With MUS a problem statement could be: 'I suffer from restless legs which is not medically explained, this lowers my mood and makes me anxious, associated with thoughts such as, this isn't fair, I can't bear these symptoms, I've got something medically wrong, I can't live my life with this. I tend to dwell on these symptoms, I avoid activity for fear of worsening them.' Possible goals with this MUS: 'I will develop a formulation that explains why I may have these symptoms; I will actively address the factors that are contributing to my symptoms. I will keep a diary to explore the link between psychological factors and my symptoms; I will not engage in medical activities for investigation or cure that do not have an evidence base; I will increase exercise and activity to build up my strength and stamina: I will do my normal activities of daily living despite my symptoms: I will be independent, and rely on others only when necessary.'

Once these statements are done and measured it is important to use them actively in the sessions, particularly if you are not using protocols but are using formulation-based approaches. In practice this would mean having them open on the table during the session, referring to them ('How does this link to the formulation?'), altering them, for example adding goals if required, measuring them at mid and end point.

## The balance between acceptance and change, when considering problems and goals

This issue is important for several reasons. One is that although with treatment, a phobia or mild depression should be overcome, one cannot cure a long-term condition, and changes in MUS may not be large. Also, recent models of therapy like ACT have put more emphasis on acceptance of difficult emotions and physical symptoms, arguing that the avoidance or resistance to symptoms creates further problems (Hayes, Strosahl & Wilson, 2011). A further complexity is that patients understandably want improvement and cure, whereas clinicians may have the view that this may not happen, so this produces a tension between acceptance and change. Our view is that with health anxiety the focus should be on change. We have good models of health anxiety and understand that catastrophic health thinking, anxious arousal and its generation of further symptoms are important maintenance factors. These factors are amenable to change and our observation is that when these change the health anxiety disappears (although it may return). With MUS we believe that change is possible: if one can find the relevant maintenance factors and change them, then there should be an improvement in symptoms, emotions, and functioning, but the improvement will not be of the size achieved with more straight-forward disorders. With long-term conditions some improvement in the condition is possible: this could be a new medication, a new medical intervention; some improvement in support like a wheelchair or walking aid. Occasionally medical progress allows the person to try to get a promising new treatment.

However, the cruel reality for many patients is that there will be no cure, their symptoms may get worse and they may die from the condition: when the patient is unable to accept, we need to consider what the best thing to do is. One thing is to consider why it may be difficult to accept the reality of LTC: it may represent uncomfortable facts about further disability and death; it may represent the end of aspirations or a sense of a life incomplete or unfulfilled; it may mean increasing acknowledgment and experience of horrible physical symptoms. The first thing is to genuinely open your heart to them: it is important to be as empathic and compassionate as possible with this tough situation they are in. If the person wants to avoid thinking about acceptance of the condition this can be difficult: particularly that they are dwelling on the condition, looking for a cure, seeking endless investigations and medical appointments. This can cause problems in that the person is not fully living their life. A goal statement here could be 'I will understand my thoughts and feelings about having this condition and consider reducing or giving up my medical consultations.' Sometimes the person is pursuing other tests, but it is a small part of their lives, and they are willing to work with you on a CBT approach. This process of adjustment may be helped by having goals (goals should always be positive), that are focused on specific valued activities: spending time with grandchildren; developing new interests; holidays that the person can pursue despite mobility problems. Some of the research on attitude in cancer patients is interesting, in that fighting spirit (seeing cancer as a challenge and developing a positive attitude) led to an improvement in quality of life (Greer et al., 1992)

What can you say to someone who as a long-term condition? Ensure that if these comments are made, they are made genuinely and with heart.

- 'Tell me what's on your mind about the condition'
- 'Tell me about your illness'
- 'It must be so hard suffering like this'
- 'Can I help you bear it more'
- 'I'll be here for you'
- 'What keeps you going?'

## Advice and discharge

If for the reasons outlined earlier, a patient is not suitable for treatment, then they are discharged after assessment. A clear explanation should be given.

- 'You are coping well without me'
- 'My heart goes out to you as to how much you are suffering but I'm not sure a CBT approach will make a difference'
- 'We can't seem to get agreement on what's causing your symptoms'

- 'Your problems are too complex or chronic for me to deal with'
- 'It seems you have other current priorities to deal with, which I completely understand'
- 'I'm not clear that psychological factors are relevant here'
- 'I'm not sure about psychological therapy whilst you are in the middle of medical treatment/investigations'

## Chapter summary

There are several generic and specific measurement tools that can be used, and it's also helpful getting patients to track links to triggers, emotions, and behaviours. Problems and goal statements are done, with careful consideration of the balance between acceptance and change. Research supports a modest effect of CBT, patients can be considered for CBT or low-intensity psychological support, or nothing.

# Part II

# Treatment approaches

Low intensity, protocol and formulation-based CBT for long-term conditions

## Chapter 4

# Low-intensity work with health conditions

In this chapter we examine the evidence base for low-intensity CBT (LICBT), present examples from practice and make suggestions how the therapist can either use LI interventions in their own practice or signpost to a PWP when working with someone with depression or anxiety with an LTC. Following the implementation of the IAPT programme in England in 2008, the stepped care model has become a defining feature of psychological services. LICBT shares the principles of CBT in that it focuses on the present, is collaborative and structured and is based on a scientific approach. One of the defining features, which sets it apart from HI CBT, is the focus on efficiency in terms of high volumes of patients and brevity of therapy course (Papworth & Marrinan, 2019). IAPT provide additional training, at both Steps 2 and 3, for working with people with LTC, and the national curriculum has been recently reviewed and updated (IAPT, 2017).

LICBT is a modern form of Behaviour Therapy, and the principal approaches used by PWPs are Behavioural Activation (BA), Exposure and habituation, worry management, Problem Solving (PS), and graded exercise. Methods go beyond face-to-face sessions, to include guided self-help which may be supported over the phone, or internet-based delivery. We will examine the main approaches here.

## Behavioural activation

Early behavioural therapy models for treating depression include the work of Lewinsohn and Shaffer (1971), and Ferster (1973) and these models promoted increased activity alone as the mechanism of change. An iconic component analysis study by Jacobson et al. (1996) made a comparison between behavioural changes alone (activity), increased activity plus cognitive restructuring, and the full CBT approach which includes changes to activity, modifying automatic negative thoughts and challenging core beliefs and rules, and no significant difference were found between the three conditions. Jacobson et al. (1996) concluded that activity alone was as effective as the other approaches for a shorter treatment course, with less training need, making it a more economical intervention. These findings have been supported repeatedly over the past two decades (Ekers, Richards & Gilbody, 2008; Richards et al., 2016). Richards et al. (2016), in a large-scale RCT

DOI: 10.4324/9780367824433-7

(commonly referred to as the COBRA study), concluded that there is no difference in outcomes for treating depression using BA or traditional CBT.

One of the first aspects to affect someone who is experiencing depression symptoms is the autonomic changes to the body's circadian rhythm. The reduction in activity and drive affect the routine markers (referred to as zeitgebers) of the person's day. This highlights the importance of targeting autonomic processes, affecting the maintenance of depression, including sleep, appetite, motivation, and concentration. Disruption to routines can have a significant impact on these processes, further affecting functioning and escalating symptoms of depression. Once symptoms increase there is then the tendency to reduce activity, which provides temporary relief through negative reinforcement. However, over time the person's daily functioning becomes increasingly affected, and the avoidance reduces opportunities for pleasure and achievement, both of which are essential for normal functioning and mood. In the absence of positive reinforcement, and continued negative reinforcement by avoidance of activity, a vicious cycle is created and maintained. To break the cycle, BA aims to regulate daily routine structures and build a balance of necessary, routine, and pleasurable activities. In pure Step 2 BA, there is no need to do a baseline activity diary if the rationale is explained appropriately. Completing the baseline diary can often add to the demands on the person, so it is seen as desirable to start planning activities based on the treatment goals set after assessment. Unlike Beck CT approaches, it does not collect hourly breakdowns of previously undertaken activity and ratings, it plans activities ahead, and patients work to the plan at those times despite difficult thoughts or symptoms. Based on the targets set, a hierarchy is built to allocate tasks according to level of difficulty. The person begins with tasks that are easier to reintroduce, and they are encouraged to focus on these until they are managed more easily over the whole week. Over time this improves mood by breaking the cycle of avoidance, and by reducing the time spent in rumination. The hierarchy helps the person to approach increasingly more taxing activities whilst reintroducing pleasurable things they have stopped doing, this provides positive reinforcement, increasing the likelihood of repeating these activities.

BA is normally delivered by a trained practitioner in order to achieve the 'treatment dose' recommended by NICE guidelines for depression (NICE, 2009). Earlier versions delivered in IAPT were developed and popularised by the collaborative headed by David Richards, who were responsible for the detailed manuals produced for LI training and practice (Richards & Whyte, 2009). A recent approach suggested by Chellingsworth (2020a) is the 'Get back to being you' booklet which is a guided self-help model. A phenomenon known as sudden gains in therapy has been highlighted by Tang, DeRubeis, Beberman and Pham (2005) in relation to CBT for depression where a person experiences a significant decrease in symptoms between one session and the next. More recently Masterson et al. (2014) have examined sudden gains in depression when using BA, and their findings support Hopko, Robertson and Carvalho (2009), who noted that BA not only produced sudden gains in nearly half of their sample of cancer patients, but that these gains were made much earlier than in traditional CBT approaches. This has implications for working with people with LTC, who may require quicker symptom relief in order to encourage engagement in therapy.

## BA for people with LTC

When considering the specific approach, BA would seem a good first line intervention for treating depression with LTC, and patients can be stepped up if required. This has been the NICE recommendation since 2009, and included in the IAPT curriculum for LICBT for LTC since the same year. Haddad (2009) commenting on the NICE guideline 'Depression in adults with a chronic physical health problem: treatment and management (NICE, 2009)' emphasised the importance of all healthcare professionals having skills in detecting depression symptoms in this population. Haddad described a two-question screening, based on the core symptoms of depression identified in longer measuring scales such as the PHQ-9. The two-question screening was proposed by Whooley, Avins, Miranda and Browner (1997) and consists of the following:

1   During the past month, have you often been bothered by feeling down, depressed, or hopeless?
2   During the past month, have you often been bothered by little interest or pleasure in doing things?

Haddad (2009) reported that this two-question screening was common in UK Primary care at the time of the NICE recommendation. Since the development of IAPT, the PHQ-9 has probably been used more widely, as a measure of depression symptoms, even by non-mental health professionals.

In practice, there are several ways that BA can help someone with LTC and depression. Table 4.1 lists some of these benefits.

*Table 4.1* Benefits of BA

| |
| --- |
| Strong evidence for the effectiveness of relieving symptoms of depression in the short-term. This is desirable for people with additional LTC who may be suffering with a range of other symptoms. |
| Generally delivered within IAPT services within 6 sessions. This can be through face-to-face or guided self-help approaches. This can be in addition to other treatments the person may be receiving for their physical health conditions. |
| Breaking the cycle of negative reinforcement (behaviours) which has been learned as a response to depressive symptoms may also be helpful regarding health-related avoidance |
| Possible to achieve some quick therapeutic gains. Raise awareness of vicious cycle and how to break it at the behavioural point. Easy to engage with. |

When it comes to empirical evidence for the use of BA for LTC, there is not a large amount of research: there was a recent Cochrane systematic review (Uphoff et al., 2020) of the use of BA in people with LTCs and they only identified two studies that met their criteria. In the review, the term non-communicable diseases (NCD) is used to describe LTC. In the review they were focusing on what WHO (2017) state as being the top four NCDs – cardiovascular disease, cancer, respiratory disease, and Type 2 diabetes. Both studies, which met the criteria for the Cochrane review, examined the use of BA to treat symptoms of depression where there was a co-morbid physical health condition. Both used an 8-week course of behavioural therapy consisting of BA. The samples used in both studies met the clinical criteria for Major Depressive Disorder (MDD) as defined in the DSM(IV-TR) (American Psychiatric Association, 2000) which was the version of the manual in use at the time of both studies. The first study was conducted by Mitchell et al. (2008). They compared BA with treatment as usual for treating depression in people recovering from a stroke. The control group received poststroke treatment as usual with no comparable depression intervention. Results showed a significant difference between the two groups in terms of recovery of depression symptoms, with the BA group recovering quicker and maintaining the therapeutic gains for longer. Hopko et al. (2011) examined the use of BA in women with breast cancer and depression. They compared BA with problem-solving sessions. Both were effective. It was their later study in 2015 (Hopko et al., 2015) that was included in the Cochrane review. Their findings highlighted some interesting issues in terms of predictors of outcomes. This is summarised in Table 4.2.

The negative effects support the findings of Driessen and Hollon (2010), who identified factors associated with overall negative treatment outcomes for MDD:

- Severity and chronicity
- Earlier age of onset of depression
- Family history of depression
- Childhood experience of maltreatment
- Co-existent psychological disorders

Table 4.2 Factors associated with outcomes

| Factors associated with favourable outcomes | Factors associated with less favourable outcomes (when receiving cancer treatment) |
| --- | --- |
| Being married or in a stable intimate relationship | Patient experiencing treatment side effects |
| Earlier experience of psychotherapy | Increased rumination, hopelessness, and worry |
| Not actively engaged in cancer treatment | Time and financial effects |

*Table 4.3* Case study BA for depression – Tanya

| | |
|---|---|
| Presentation | Tanya is 46 years old and was diagnosed with Fibromyalgia two years ago. She has chronic pain and has experienced symptoms of depression and anxiety for the past 6 months. She has not previously been involved with mental health services. The pain is being managed with over-the-counter pain relief. The depression and anxiety symptoms have caused vast fluctuations in their level of activity each day: limited activity when client is in pain and high levels of activity when the pain is manageable. The unpredictability of not knowing how they will feel physically in the upcoming days will trigger the client to worry and therefore they will avoid doing activities believing that it will make the pain worse. Initial scores: PHQ-9 = 19, GAD-7 = 17 indicating severe symptoms of depression and anxiety. |
| Brief historical background | Prior to the diagnosis Tanya has always been a high achiever, works hard and is very driven. No previous episodes of depression or noticeable anxiety were present. |
| Problem statement | 'My main problem is trying to manage the symptoms of Fibromyalgia. This is triggered by everyday things such as, washing the pots and taking my son to school. When this happens, I think How am I going to feel tomorrow? and What if I cannot take my son to school? At times like this my body responds with tiredness, tension, aches and pains. When all this happens, I respond by becoming less motivated and I will struggle to get out of bed. This is a problem because I have stopped doing the things I enjoy.' |
| Goals | 1 To not worry about how I am going to feel the next day<br>2 To be able to start swimming and walking again<br>3 To be able to concentrate better to start reading and doing puzzles again |
| Treatment | **Behavioural Activation** with pacing to help manage the symptoms of Fibromyalgia, and to work towards the patient's goals of going swimming and walking, and of doing reading and puzzle activities.<br>Some adaptations were agreed by patient, practitioner and supervisor to overcome barriers:<br>• to use simplified worksheets rather than detailed booklets<br>• to have longer sessions of 45 minutes that were slower-paced<br>• to incorporate pacing breaks to help manage the patient's difficulties with poor concentration during sessions<br>**Worry Management** was also used as the patient was still experiencing hypothetical worries relating to future flare ups of Fibromyalgia. |
| Outcomes | The patient engaged well throughout treatment and after five sessions she reported feeling much better in mood, had achieved all her goals and her scores were sub-clinical:<br>PHQ-9 = 6<br>GAD-7 = 6 |

At the time of writing, there are feasibility studies being conducted in order to meet the criteria for a randomised controlled trial to evaluate the effectiveness of BA for people who have had a stroke (Thomas et al., 2019). In their study group, BEADS (which stands for Behavioural Activation for Depression in Stroke), they have found that BA is acceptable to patients, their carers and services, but it is still early in the research programme to conclude how effective BA is for this patient group long term and what, if any, specific issues may apply.

## Exposure and habituation

At Step 2, one of the principal approaches for treating anxiety is exposure therapy. This is taught in the IAPT curriculum and is based on learning theory. Exposure therapy is used for treating panic disorder, specific phobias, and agoraphobia, which could be present in the person with an LTC. The mechanism of change in exposure therapy is the extinction of fear, by habituation to the feared stimuli, and this is achieved by breaking the cycle of avoidance that reinforces the fear. Exposure and habituation therapy begins with clear psycho-education to explain the physiological response to fear that is triggered in panic disorder, specific phobia, and agoraphobia. The vicious cycle is then used to show how the trigger becomes conditioned by the repetitive use of safety and avoidance behaviours, which reinforces the level of threat associated with the trigger. Thus, when the person avoids the trigger, they fail to learn it is not dangerous.

Care needs to be taken, when working with people with LTC, to fully understand the symptom profile of their physical health condition. This can be explored by the use of a symptom diary to record physical sensations in context. For example, by asking the person to state the physical sensation/symptom, when it occurred, and what emotional reaction they experienced, it is useful in terms of separating out a symptom that occurs regardless of anxiety. In their study of non-cardiac chest pain, Marks, Chambers, Russell and Hunter (2016) found that a Step 2 LICBT approach was helpful for symptom reduction through clear psych-education including self-help information on exposure and habituation to avoided triggers. This was a clinical evaluation study so no control group was used for comparison, and little detail was provided in terms of specific interventions used, but findings indicate that guided self-help is useful for this client group. This is supported by a recent pilot study of Step 2 LICBT interventions for non-cardiac chest pain at an Emergency Department (ED) in Australia (Wilkinson et al., 2019). There was a significant decrease in re-presentation to ED bringing about a saving to the healthcare provider.

In the evidence-based Step 2 booklet 'Fears conquered with exposure and habituation', Chellingsworth (2020b), sets out a clear step-by-step patient guide, to be facilitated by a trained professional (normally a PWP). Beginning with the explanation of the fear response and maintenance cycle, there follows the creation of a hierarchy of feared situations and triggers to develop a coherent treatment plan, the active exposure and habituation treatment phase, and relapse prevention.

Examples of this are gradual exposure to agoraphobic situations such as crowds, being far from home and activity. If there is complexity or risk the patient should be stepped up (see Chapter 6).

## Worry management using PMR, and worry time

The LICBT approaches for managing worry normalises worry and stress as a part of everyday life. This is appealing for someone with an LTC, as worry can be normalised in the context of their condition and treatment is not complex. In Chellingsworth's (2020c) 'Worry less, live more with GAD' approach, the following stages are presented: psychoeducation on the cycle of worry, progressive muscle relaxation to reduce tension and raise awareness of the physiological impact of worry, and classifying worries as problems or hypothetical worries. A designated time for addressing worries (known as 'worry time') is used and this postpones the worries rather than continuously engaging with them throughout the day. In the allotted worry time, the person is encouraged to distinguish between problems that need action or attention and hypothetical worries.

Progressive muscle relaxation (PMR) is a change method recommended in clinical guidelines for GAD and insomnia, and has been used for other conditions. It is also widely used to manage anxiety in cancer treatment (Baider, Uziely & Kaplan De-Nour, 1994; Pelekasis, Matsouka & Koumarionou, 2017), IBS and other health conditions. By getting the person to focus their attention on each muscle group as they go through the exercise, they are encouraged to maintain a present-moment focus. PMR also helps with the secondary symptoms associated with tension, including pain, headaches, irritability, and sleep problems. The procedure involves tensing each muscle set for five seconds then releasing the tension. A script can be followed as given in the subsequent text (Chellingsworth, 2020c).

My forehead: lift my eyebrows as high as I can, and tense.
My face: tighten up the muscles in my face, around my cheeks and nose and
    hold it tense.
My jaw: hold my jaw slightly open and tense it.
My neck: gently lean my head right back, stretching my neck and hold it tense
My shoulders: lift my shoulders to my neck and tense.
My upper back: push my arms backwards at chest level, with elbows towards
    each other
My right arm at the top: tighten my bicep muscle and tense it as if showing
    someone my muscles.
My left arm at the top: repeat as previously said with my left bicep muscle.
My right hand and forearm: make a fist and tense my lower arm and stretch it
    out, keeping it tense.
My left hand and forearm: repeat the previous one with my left hand and
    forearm.

My upper back and shoulder blades: stretch up my back and shoulder blades, and hold them tense.

My abdomen and lower back: pull in my tummy muscles and hold them tight and tense. My buttocks: tighten my buttocks, and tense them up.

My entire right leg: put my leg out and tense it all the way down. My entire left leg: repeat the previous one on my left side.

My lower right leg and calf: tense my calf muscle in my lower leg. My lower left leg and calf: repeat the previous one with my left side.

My right foot: curl up my toes and tense my foot. My left foot: repeat the previous step with my left foot.

The muscle is tensed for five seconds then released for five seconds.

Following the PMR, the patient is shown how to classify worries into actual problems or hypothetical worries. If it is a problem then problem-solving techniques can be taught and encouraged (see the next section), but if hypothetical then worry time is encouraged. Worry time is defined by Chellingsworth (2020c, p. 9) as 'an effective strategy to manage worries more effectively and reduce affect, to decrease worry being interpreted as a helpful strategy, and increase aversion through paradoxical intention (deliberate worrying during worry time)'. The patient sets a planned time to worry. During other times they are encouraged to write any worries down and bring attention back to the present. At the designated time they can revisit the worries they recorded in the day. Once the worry time ends, they should destroy the list of worries and start the process again. It is an effective strategy and one that could be helpful for people with LTC to allow them a time to worry without it impacting throughout the entire day (Borkovec, Shadick & Hopkins, 1991)

## Problem solving

Problem Solving (PS) is a fundamental skill taught at both Step 2 and Step 3 as a means for helping people to overcome avoidance when experiencing symptoms of depression and/or anxiety. Helping the person to recognise the difference between actual problems that require their attention and action, and hypothetical worries (of a 'what if?' type) which may not have a resolution, is a vital first step.

That patients have difficulties with problem solving in relation to worry, have been recognised since the early work of Borkovec et al. (1983), and in his influential paper (Borkovec, 1985) cognitive avoidance is seen as the mechanism by which worry impacts on problem solving. If the person is trying to avoid thinking about their perceived 'problems', then they are less likely to address them, which actually further increases their worry and avoidance. D'Zurilla and Nezu (1982) distinguished between problem orientation and problem solving, suggesting that worry impairs the person in identifying the specific problem in the first instance. Dugas and Robichaud (2007) in their Intolerance of uncertainty CBT model, support these two processes, suggesting that people who worry excessively are no worse at solving problems, but the worry acts as a barrier to identifying and addressing (or orientating to) the problem in the first place.

In her Step 2 approach Chellingsworth (2020c) uses the problem-solving strategies espoused in the earlier work of Borkovec.

1   Turn the worry into a practical problem – what do I need to do, and when do I need to do it by?
2   List as many workable solutions to the problem (not matter how silly they may seem, don't discount any)
3   Do a 'pros' and 'cons' for each potential solution
4   Choose one of the solutions and write a plan of how you are going to carry it out
5   Do it
6   Evaluate it – how did it go? Do I need to revise it or try another potential solution?

In terms of applying problem-solving strategies with people with LTC, Fitzpatrick, Schumann and Hill-Briggs (2013) examined problem solving in the self-management of diabetes in a systematic review examining 16 intervention studies. They found no significant effect when compared to control groups, although there was great variance in terms of individual study designs and problem solving was one of many strategies that were identified as being helpful in the self-management of diabetes. However, Malouff, Thorsteinsson and Schutte (2007) found that PS across-the-board had a beneficial effect on psychological and physical disorders, better than no treatment, and equal to equivalent treatments.

## Self-help methods

LICBT has used guided self-help as a principal tool for applying CBT at a Step 2 level. The IAPT curriculum was built around comprehensive evidence-based guides for teaching PWPs how to deliver guided self-help (Richards & Whyte, 2011). This method of delivery is one of the features of LICBT that makes it efficient and accessible to a wide range of people. CBT has always had a self-help principle at its core, so the development of methods that go beyond just face-to-face therapist delivery is also clearly more cost-effective (Hughes, Herron & Younge, 2014). Other benefits include:

•   The patient has quick access to interventions that work.
•   They can work at their own pace.
•   Information materials and sources are always available for reference or relapse prevention.

Self-help CBT treatment can incorporate different methods of delivery including bibliotherapy (manuals and reading materials), telephone, computer, applications on mobile phones or via the internet. The efficacy of the different methods is hard to generalise but a number of studies suggest that outcomes are significantly higher when the self-help material is accompanied by a skilled and supportive practitioner (Gellatly et al., 2007; Spek et al., 2007). Important considerations include: how easy the material is to understand; how closely it reflects the original evidence-based CBT protocol; skill level of the practitioner; how much input is needed by the practitioner to optimise outcomes; and how effective the management of the delivery is, from an organisational perspective, to ensure clinical governance.

Bibliotherapy refers to a range of written materials often presented in manualised form, for the delivery of evidence-based protocols. This includes Behavioural Activation (BA) for depression, and manuals that support the treatment of anxiety disorders (see, e.g. the CBT Resource at www.thecbtresource.co.uk). One of the most comprehensive self-help packages, which incorporates bibliotherapy and internet-based methods with on-line support is Living Life to the Full (LLTTF) developed by Chris Williams (www.llttf.com). He has also produced a series of structured self-help workbooks using the Five Areas approach (Williams & Chellingsworth, 2010) consistent with traditional CBT. Initially providing resources targeting depression and anxiety, the programme has developed to include a much broader range of presenting problems and client groups including LTCs. At time of writing three packages are available: Living Life to the Full for Chronic Pain; Living Life to the Full for Diabetes, and Reclaim Your Life. The core modules are provided free, with additional support and resources with registration.

Computerised CBT (cCBT) was developed over 30 years ago, with a classic study by Selmi (1990) showing that CBT delivered by an interactive computer program on CD-ROM was as effective as therapist delivered CBT. Computer-based CBT has evolved considerably since the inception of the IAPT programme. Andersson (2009) highlights the leading role the internet plays in modern life in the developed world, and as such provides a familiar format that can in most cases reduce the threat associated with seeking therapy. Andrews et al. (2018) conducted a meta-analysis of 64 RCTs, examining the effectiveness of internet-based CBT (iCBT) and Computerised CBT (cCBT) against control groups, and found both to be effective in treating major depression, panic disorder, social phobia, and generalised anxiety disorder. In nine of the studies, results were shown to be comparable to face-to-face delivery. Chikersal et al. (2020) highlight problems with engagement and attrition on internet therapy platforms. They found in their study that integrating a human supporter increases engagement and clinical outcomes. This was achieved by providing concrete, positive, and supportive feedback with reference to social behaviours. In addition to iCBT, there are a number of applications available to use on mobile phones to support LICBT self-help approaches. One such app is based on the self-help protocol for Irritable Bowel Syndrome (IBS) developed by Hunt (2016).

Clearly the materials and resources listed in Table 4.4 would be useful to anyone presenting with depression or anxiety in addition to an LTC. In addition to these, there are LICBT approaches that have been specifically adapted to meet the

*Table 4.4* Some of the common self-help resources available currently in the UK

| Type of self-help material | Examples | Comments |
| --- | --- | --- |
| Bibliotherapy (evidence-based manualised materials) | IAPT Reach Out student materials https://cedar.exeter.ac.uk/ | Comprehensive curriculum training manuals for PWPs, describing in detail how to deliver guided self-help at Step 2. |
| | The CBT Resource www.cbtresource.co.uk | Provides self-help materials, worksheets, clinician protocols and guides. These materials are available for individual use only, free with paid annual subscription. |
| | 'Overcoming' book series | A series of self-help books presenting evidence-based CBT for a range of mental health problems including depression, different types of anxiety disorders and low self-esteem. They are also available as part of the Books on Prescription scheme in the UK, whereby patients can access these guides via their local library. |
| | Anxiety Canada www.anxietycanada.ca | Free downloadable informati on booklets and worksheets on a range of anxiety disorders, using a CBT perspective. |
| | Centre for Clinical Investigations (CCI) www.cci.health.wa.gov.au | Australian Psychology organisation, supported by the Government health Department, that provides free clinical resources in line with evidence-based psychological therapy, mainly from a CBT perspective. In addition to self-help materials there is updated information on latest research. |
| Internet based CBT (iCBT) models | Living Life to the Full (LLTTF) www.llttf.com | A range of topics based on the 5 areas approach. Many packages are free, with additional modules available for subscription. Books are also available to buy, or on the 'Books on Prescription' scheme. |

*(Continued)*

*Table 4.4* (Continued)

| Type of self-help material | Examples | Comments |
| --- | --- | --- |
| | Silvercloud www.silvercloud.com | Digital health provider system. Over 30 programmes across the spectrum of mental health problems. Used routinely in many IAPT services to support Step 2 practice. |
| | Omnitherapy.org | NHS funded resource for anyone over the age of 17 in the Leeds area. Video courses on a range of issues: depression and anxiety, stress, self-esteem, post-natal depression, and bereavement |
| | Regul8 | A web-based CBT self-management programme, developed by Chalder, Windgassen, Sibelli, Burgess and Moss-Morris (2014) in partnership with patients |
| Applications (Apps) | Zemedy 2 – IBS app www.zemedy.com | Based on self-help protocol for irritable bowel syndrome (IBS) developed by Hunt, Ertel, Coello and Rodriguez (2015). Zemedy 2 is the updated version, which has been released in 2020. |
| | Mindshift www.anxietycanada.com | App produced by Anxiety Canada, aimed at helping people to understand and manage their symptoms with information and tools that are compatible with a CBT model. |
| | NHS apps series www.nhs.uk/apps-library/ category/mental-health/ | A range of mental health related apps supported and endorsed by the NHS in UK. Content may change according to recommendations at the time of searching. |

needs of people with LTC. Hadert (2013) provides a systematic review on adapting guided self-help for people with LTC. She suggests that adaptations are most effective when: they recognise the interaction between the LTC and anxiety or depression; address illness-related cognitions that contribute to excess disability; and adjusting expectations to increase re-engagement in valued activities. In addition to self-help for people with LTC, there has been research to show that it can also help those caring for someone with an LTC. For example, the work of Woodford and Richards is aimed at informal carers of stroke survivors, and compares supported cognitive behavioural self-help with treatment as usual. This is at the feasibility for RCT stage of the research programme, and a recent summary suggests difficulties with recruitment (Farrand, 2020), so more conclusive findings will be forthcoming.

## Graded exercise

It is widely recognised that exercise is good for both physical and mental well-being (La Forge et al., 1999), but it is only more recently that research evidence has identified the specific factors and mechanisms of change responsible for these effects (Rethorst, Landers, Nagoshi & Ross, 2010). In the NICE (2009) guidelines for 'Depression in adults with a chronic health condition', guidance for interventions, aimed at increasing physical activity, at each step are provided. For Step 2 it recommends group activity sessions spanning over 12–14 sessions, ideally two or three sessions per week. Indeed, the Department of Health (2011) 4-year plan for developing talking therapies, for people with long-term physical health problems, also endorsed this recommendation.

The autonomic changes that occur when someone is experiencing symptoms of depression causes a disruption to the balance of chemicals responsible for mood regulation. Exercise is known for the increase in endorphins, which can give an experience of pleasure and satisfaction, but it also has many other neuropsychological effects (Rethorst et al., 2010). These include:

- Monoamines – serotonin/nor-adrenaline increase similar to SSRIs/SNRIs
- Impact on cortisol release – down-regulates the sympathetic nervous system (reducing symptoms)
- Increased body temperature – physical relaxation effect
- Refocus of attention away from rumination
- Improved cognitive performance

As part of an adapted Step 2 intervention for people with Type 2 diabetes mellitus (T2DM), Wroe, Rennie, Gibbons, Hassy and Chapman (2015); Wroe, Rennie, Sollesse and Chapman (2018) emphasised the importance of exercise to minimise symptoms of anxiety and depression, and there was a marked increase in physical activity in this group by the end of the six-week group intervention. Feedback from the study group suggested that this message had been acted upon within the BA element of the programme.

Carter, Morres, Meade and Callaghan (2016) have examined the effect of exercise on adolescents with mental health problems of varying degrees. Their findings suggest significant improvement in mood when exercise is encouraged and maintained. They highlight the importance of the exercise being meaningful and pleasurable, although it is the engagement in the physical activity itself which is believed to produce the positive effects. If we accept that the target group in these studies are complex, varied and traditionally difficult to engage, then we should expect that these findings could be realised by other patient groups with similar complexity. In the case of people with a co-morbid physical and mental health problem, for example difficulties with engagement and motivation, due to chronic avoidance, are also likely to be barriers to exercise.

## Chapter summary

This chapter has provided an overview of the LICBT approach to treating depression and anxiety, and how it can be used when working with someone with an LTC. Several resources are available to support treatment, and being flexible in your approach is vital in order to offer choice and variety and increase engagement in psychological therapy. LICBT can help the person feel more in control of their mental health recovery by offering a broader self-help approach to symptom management. Research is limited in terms of conclusive evidence around CBT for LTC, at both Steps 2 and 3, but there are some large-scale studies in the process and the evidence in general for the LICBT is strong enough to guide clinical practice.

## Chapter 5

# Cognitive therapy for depression in long-term conditions

In this chapter we will consider how depression can be understood and treated, from a CBT high intensity perspective, when there is a co-morbid LTC. It is assumed that as cognitive behavioural therapists, the reader already has a working knowledge of the fundamental CBT knowledge and skills necessary to treat depression. However, in order to provide a clear context for working with this patient group, we will review some of the main tenets of both Cognitive Science and Learning Theory which inform the evidence base for CBT treatment for depression. Here we are describing the treatment of clinical depression: this is to disentangle it from a normal adjustment reaction that will occur if a person develops an LTC. So, in depression the person has a host of symptoms including tiredness, poor sleep, lack of enjoyment in life that is impacting on his life over and above the LTC. Sometimes there can be an attributional belief such as 'having an illness is making me depressed' thus the depression is ascribed to the medical condition, and it needs to be remembered that not all patients who experience chronic ill health are depressed.

Behavioural activation has been described in the last chapter so in this chapter we will provide a brief overview of the development of CBT through what have become known as the three 'waves'. We will describe a Beckian Cognitive Therapy (CT) approach to depression and examine the use of imagery work for depression in LTC. The more recent Third Wave approaches that draw on notions of acceptance, tolerance and compassion are discussed in the following chapter. The message throughout this book is that we need to be open and creative as to how we can, not only adapt existing protocols for depression and anxiety disorders for people with LTC, but also look beyond these and consider approaches from other areas of the spectrum of CBT theoretical positions.

## Three waves of CBT development and their relevance to depression and LTC

### First wave – behaviourism

This is often viewed as the earliest form of CBT, or the first wave. There is an emphasis on reinforcement as the mechanism of change. Schwartz and Beatty

DOI: 10.4324/9780367824433-8

(1977) developed the bio-feedback technique, which led to an interest in the interaction between physical health and mental health in terms of psychological response to physical symptoms. This was influential in the development of the discipline of Behavioural Medicine, which expanded psychopathological understandings of mental health problems in terms of a bio-psychosocial perspective. Fast forwarding to the present day, BT is still widely used. It has become one of the most popular approaches to treating mild to moderate mental health problems as a Step 2 intervention. Chapter 4 outlines how this approach can be used to treat people with depression and an LTC in more detail.

### Second wave – cognitions and information processing

Beck (1985) developed a style of delivering therapy where the therapist and the patient work in collaboration on a journey of guided discovery. Socratic questioning is designed to help the person make links between their beliefs and behaviours and how these patterns affect their emotions. Theories and hypotheses can be tested using experiments between sessions as homework tasks. Beck identified three levels of cognition: core beliefs which are formed in early life and are rigidly held as truths; rules for living which serve to minimise the activation of the core beliefs; and Negative Automatic Thoughts (NATs) which are activated in specific contexts and are associated with the core beliefs. A key aspect of Beck's cognitive model of depression is what is termed the negative cognitive triad (Beck, Rush, Shaw & Emery, 1979). This refers to three specific themes that describe the content of depression related automatic negative thoughts. These three themes are: negative view of self, 'I am useless'; negative view of the world, 'The world is harsh'; and negative view of the future, 'Everything is pointless'. Treatment includes activity scheduling, challenging thoughts and rules for living, through behavioural experiments.

The table should help you decide which approach best fits the presenting problem, needs and goals of the person. It is not always the case that complexity determines the treatment approach although NICE guidelines suggest trying behavioural approaches for more mild-to-moderate depressive symptoms.

Let us look in more detail at how depression can be treated with the Beck CT approach.

## Cognitive therapy for depression with an LTC

When considering people with LTC and depression, a cognitive therapy approach would aim to understand the onset and development of beliefs that have made them vulnerable to depression. This includes their past experiences and beliefs about illness, and what illness behaviours these experiences have resulted in. We are assuming that the reader is already familiar with and skilled in delivering cognitive interventions for people presenting with depression, so we just want to highlight how these skills can be honed for people with an LTC.

*Table 5.1* Comparison of CT for depression approach with Behavioural Activation (BA)

|  | Cognitive therapy for depression | Behavioural activation |
| --- | --- | --- |
| Theoretical position | Negative thinking biases are present in depression and are associated with the activation of negative core beliefs developed in earlier life. Rumination on these negative beliefs is a major maintenance factor in depression.<br>Three levels of cognition (NATs, rules and core beliefs) are interrelated and implicated in how people behave both when depressed and not. | When people become depressed a cycle of avoidance is set up, which becomes negatively reinforced as stopping doing things initially provided relief. Over time, the reduction of activities maintains the depressed mood as there is a lack of pleasure and sense of achievement, and a disruption to routines. Based on Learning theory. |
| Evidence base | The most researched approach within CBT. Some consistency in findings which have influenced clinical guidelines, but still a lack of strong evidence across all conditions and for long-term recovery from symptoms | Strong evidence for the effectiveness of relieving symptoms of depression in the short-term. Difficulties in separating out if the behavioural changes alone produce symptom relief. |
| NICE recommended treatment length | Traditionally recommended 12–20 sessions in line with Beck's original protocol. | Generally delivered within IAPT services within six sessions. This can be through face-to-face or guided self-help approaches. |
| Mechanism of change | Modification of dysfunctional beliefs through testing and updating. Experiments involve changing behaviours to test the predictions (beliefs) held by the person. | Breaking the cycle of negative reinforcement (behaviours) which has been learned as a response to depressive symptoms. |
| Strengths of model for LTC & MUS | Highlighting beliefs that may not have been in the person's awareness due to cognitive and emotional avoidance which is characteristic of these presentations.<br>Reducing rumination through modifying unhelpful beliefs may have a longer-term impact than just breaking the cycle. | Possible to achieve some quick therapeutic gains. Raise awareness of vicious cycle and how to break it at the behavioural point. Easy to engage with. |

*(Continued)*

*Table 5.1* (Continued)

|  | Cognitive therapy for depression | Behavioural activation |
|---|---|---|
| Challenges of approach for LTC & MUS | Cognitive processes may interfere with engagement – i.e. working with the thoughts may trigger more distress in the short-term, which would risk disengagement. May not resonate with the person's understanding of their problems. Fatigue and pain may be barriers to working at a cognitive level. | Lack of opportunities to change some of the necessary, routine and pleasurable behaviours due to chronic pain, mobility problems or fatigue. |

Beck cognitive therapy for depression treatment planning

- Assessment of presenting problems within a CBT framework including socialisation to the CBT model (1–3 sessions)
- Problem and target setting (1 session)
- Behavioural intervention: activity scheduling and graded task assignment (3–6 sessions)
- Cognitive intervention: attentional focus strategies; counting thoughts and TICS (therapy interfering cognitions) and TOCS (therapy orienting cognitions) Burns (2012) (1–2 sessions)
- Cognitive behavioural intervention: identifying negative automatic thoughts; modifying automatic negative thoughts and behavioural experiments; tackling psychological/situational problems (4–6 sessions)
- Relapse prevention: identifying conditional beliefs; modifying conditional beliefs and behavioural experiments; managing setbacks; blueprints for change (2–4 sessions)

### The formulation of loss

The specific contribution made by Beck is to differentiate between actual and perceived loss in relation to depression. Actual losses may include loss of health; loss of ability to work or look after home and family; loss of time for leisure and enjoyment; possible loss of normal lifespan because of the health condition. Beck develops this theme further by considering the perceived losses that may accompany these actual losses. These perceived losses might include loss of purpose, loss of status, loss of role, loss of security or loss of companionship and the like. The drawing of this distinction highlights a central feature of the cognitive model, namely it is not events in themselves that make us happy, sad, angry, guilty, but the view that we take of them, regarding the loss event. For people with LTC there are some clear actual losses, such as health, financial and relationships due to symptoms and disability, but it is important that we consider the interpretation of these losses on the person's beliefs about self, others and the world. For example, if a person is presenting with depression and has been diagnosed with cancer, they will be experiencing changes in health that may lead to stopping work. These changes can be considered as actual losses – health and work – but there may be additional perceived losses such as loss of role as provider for the family, or strong protector which are now viewed as absent. These losses may be as distressing as the actual losses so it is important that they are fully explored during assessment and formulated clearly. The theme of hopelessness is a crucial aspect of depression and is related to the third theme in the Negative Cognitive Triad, a negative view of the future.

Hopelessness is defined as: 'A perception that the future is bleak and will remain so for the foreseeable future.' Of course, in this situation of having a chronic medical condition, then one's future may be limited and filled with foreboding, so the task of the therapist is to focus on helping the patient in living a full, valuable and enjoyable life whilst suffering a chronic illness, not always easy. The theme of helplessness may be present and this has emerged from the work of Seligman and Beagley (1975), and is defined as: 'a perception that there is no action an individual can take to influence a given set of circumstances'.

### Activity scheduling and graded task assignment

Within the early stages of implementation of the treatment protocol for acute depression there is an active and deliberate targeting of depressive symptoms. Tackling these first can often lead to a rapid improvement in mood over 2–6 sessions. The first intervention, after the assessment session, and to tackle depressive symptoms is the introduction of activity scheduling and graded task assignment (Beck et al., 1979; Fennell, 1999). A diary is initially kept of mastery and pleasure: this is a useful homework task in order to gain a baseline measure of the current activity levels.

*Table 5.2* Troubleshooting problems with activity scheduling

| Potential problem | Suggested solutions |
| --- | --- |
| Break things down into small chunks | For example, if the person wants to tackle the housework, then this could be broken down into doing 30 minutes a day, or doing 15 minutes of housework, then having a rest. This should be done collaboratively with the patient. TOCs such as 'this is pathetic . . . I used to do so much more . . . it'll never get done' need to be addressed. |

*(Continued)*

*Table 5.2* (Continued)

| Potential problem | Suggested solutions |
|---|---|
| Patient should pace themselves | • the rationale for this is that the person should not be doing so much that they risk a significant exacerbation of their symptoms, or they become avoidant and do nothing, or they get in to a boom-and-bust attitude, cycling between overdoing it feeling exhausted and in pain, and giving up. This is a common pattern that is easy to get into, as one can explain, and an activity schedule can be planned that attempts to iron that out. There are several ways to do this; typically, we would ask that the patient have a balance between activities that are tiring and those that are more energy giving. We could ask the patient to do a schedule of activities that start low in a way that they do not worsen symptoms, and gradually increase them. Occasionally patients are overactive, often tiring themselves and worsening symptoms, this is likely to be associated with thoughts such as 'this will not beat me'. |
| Making allowances for symptoms and depression and physical illness symptoms. | • This may manifest itself in patients downplaying the impact of their symptoms, but then feeling defeated when they are unable to do the AS. So, when planning this it is important to be realistic and set the task as 'difficult but do-able' the person can be encouraged to use TOCS such as 'I can try something . . . this will be tougher because of my problems but I can do it . . . if I can't do all I planned I can do something' |
| Making allowances for the fact that the person just may not be able to do earlier activities | • These may be enjoyable activities, or even housework or basic activities of daily living like washing, dressing, walking, making food, etc. One choice is to seek help or consider moving to a residence in which help is more easily available. Alternatively, one can say, 'Even although you are not able to do this is there some new activity that you could do that you would enjoy or value'. Examples may be things that are not very active such as: computer, internet, reading, audiobooks, sewing, crafts, etc. |
| Enlisting help and support to do activities | This could come from a partner, child, friend, voluntary group, etc. The problem here may be that for the person who has been very independent and who values autonomy and independence, this may be difficult and elicit a lot of NATS. Occasionally this can work the other way and patients become dependent on aid in circumstances in which they could do something independently. |
| Feeling judged for being ill, looking different, and not looking after self | • A lot of patients will worry about these things, there may be some reality in them. This sense of being judged could discourage them from leaving the house and engaging in things. |
| Mortality and meaning | Patient may become pre-occupied with this, or may downplay it and deny it in way that prevent them having a full life. |

As part of the activity scheduling, it is important to help patients manage their actual symptoms and get the most out of the health system. Here are some things that can be worked on, after the basics have been achieved (Uslan, 2003):

- Gaining and maintaining the support of their General Practitioner and physicians, preparing for meeting with them and having goals in mind. Deciding whether to participate in trials of new treatments
- Ensuring medication use is effective: accessing it, and being on the right drugs
- Gaining help in adjusting lifestyle, for example making practical changes to the house and car, which make them easier to use. The Occupational Therapist may be able to advise on this.
- Eating well, exercising and maintaining general health
- Using electronic aides such as mobile phones and 'tablets', to aid memory and concentration problems
- Attending and contributing to support groups and advocacy groups
- Getting the most of being in the disabled category, for example travelling provisions, work-rehabilitation, 'Expert patient program'
- Getting the most out of alternative medicine approaches

## Working with NATS in LTC

Following the activity scheduling phase of the CT model of depression is a focus on thought work. We recommend that you use thought diaries in line with Beck's CT for depression to help the person recognise and challenge NATs where appropriate. There are some special issues, however, in relation to NATs associated with LTC. The issue that arises is that patients with long-term health problems may have what could be called realistic NATS, and the best approaches are as presented in Table 5.3.

Another approach is more radical acceptance of the situation. Aspects of not accepting it may be, avoiding taking about it, downplaying the seriousness of the symptoms, seeking treatments that will not have any effect, seeking a cure, investing heavily in alternative treatments. This is a complex issue: if a patient is avoiding the issue consider what the pros and cons are of encouraging him to face it. One's natural feeling is that things like this should not be avoided, but can it beneficial if they are? Feifel, Strack and Nagy (1987) found that choice of coping strategies was influenced by personality and situational factors, that anger and confrontation was surprisingly common. Here it was found that avoidance of what they called 'Acceptance/resignation' was a helpful strategy in non-life-threatening conditions but less so in more severe disorders. Murberg, Furze and Bru (2004) showed that avoidant coping styles in congestive heart failure led to increased mortality at six years. This was primarily

*Table 5.3* Working with NATS in LTC

| Approach | Description |
|---|---|
| Work out aspects of the thought that is not true | If the person says, 'I've been told that my walking will deteriorate, I'm just going to be a burden' one could respond 'that sounds really tough that your walking will deteriorate, but does that mean you will be a burden' |
| Be as empathic and compassionate as possible | One could spend time thinking how one would react if you were unable to walk, how would you feel, what would you think, what a loss it would be. The therapist should try to feel that emotional connection to another human being who is in such a difficult predicament. It can be difficult for patients to be self-compassionate and this may be associated with thoughts such as 'I need to be strong . . . always fight it . . . don't be weak . . . I've got myself into this mess.' One can just try to show self-compassion through touch, words and a caring attitude. |
| Reversal activity | Taylor (2006) has the good suggestion of a 'reversal activity': the patient should take an action to reverse the maladaptive mood. These could be coping mechanisms; self-care activities; gratifying activities; distraction activities; pleasurable activities; motivation activities; goal orientated activities. The patient is encouraged to create and carry with them a list of specific activities from these categories that they can use if they are unable to address the negative thought. |
| Gratitude or benefit-finding | This needs to be handled sensitively to prevent the patient feeling that their suffering is not being properly acknowledged. So, the patient can be asked to respond by asking 'is there any possible learning (or benefit) that can come out of this difficult situation?' Or 'despite this thought being true is there anything that I can be grateful for now?', often this strategy works better with the homework of writing down (1, 2 or 3) things each day that the patient is grateful for. |

through the mechanism of behavioural disengagement. Regarding cancer, coping through social support, focusing on the positive and distancing were associated with less emotional distress; use of cognitive and behavioural escape/avoidance was associated with more emotional distress (Dunkel-Schetter, Feinstein, Taylor and Falke, 1992).

In summary, we have highlighted the main features of Beck's CT for depression model and how they relate and can be adapted when working with people with LTC. Table 5.4 summarises these.

*Table 5.4* CT skills in LTC

| CBT skill | Focus for LTC |
|---|---|
| Thought challenging | Recognising and changing NATs in present situations triggered by their health conditions. This may be related to functioning or reactions to pain or fatigue (e.g. 'I can't do it,' 'I'm useless'). |
| Behavioural experiments | There will be many NATs that can be tested using behavioural experiments. Constructing the belief as a 'if . . . then' statement makes it easier to test. As earlier, these may be related to predictions regarding:<br>• perceived consequences of doing certain activities (e.g. 'if I do any housework my pain will get worse').<br>• Fear of what others think of them (e.g. 'if I express how I am feeling, then I will be rejected') |
| Working with rules | The most common rule present in people with LTC is likely to be the 'all or nothing' rule. This is one of the most rigid beliefs which leads to a swing between over activity and avoidance, what has become known as the 'boom and bust' style of activity. |

To tie the elements of working with depression with an LTC the following case study demonstrates how an open and flexible approach looks like.

*Table 5.5* Case study – John

| | |
|---|---|
| Presentation | John is a 42-year-old man who was diagnosed with Type 1 diabetes, two years ago. This followed an 18-month period of feeling unwell and not knowing why. Since his diagnosis he has found it difficult to maintain activities he used to enjoy, and due to prolonged periods of sickness he decided to leave his job as a coach driver.<br>His mood has been noticeably low to his wife and family for several months, and recently he became so low that he had suicidal thoughts. This scared him into seeking help. |
| Brief historical background | John has been reasonably healthy throughout his life. When he was 12 years old his father had a mild heart attack, after which he never worked again. Illness was treated very seriously with his mum insisting that he take time off school with any minor symptom such as aches or pains. He does not recall going to hospital as a child or even visiting the GP very much, as his parents didn't trust doctors and preferred to manage by themselves. |
| Maintenance Formulation | Going through a recent example of when he felt low, the following formulation was developed:<br>Situation – sat in the conservatory watching his children playing football in the garden<br>Physical sensations – heart rate slightly raised, fatigue, tension<br>Emotions – sadness<br>Thoughts – I should be playing with them, I am a bad dad, I am useless, things are going to get worse, what's the point<br>Behaviours – stayed in the conservatory for several hours<br>This shows the excessive rumination and negative thoughts associated with his perceived loss of activity. |

*(Continued)*

*Table 5.5* (Continued)

| | |
|---|---|
| Key cognitions | From examining the historical information, we formulated the following key beliefs:<br>Core beliefs – I am weak (developed in response to illness)<br>Rules – If I can't perform 100%, then there is no point in doing it (all or nothing)<br>This makes sense of his response to work, believing that his illness will prevent him from functioning, therefore quitting his job. |
| Goals | - To reduce rumination by 50% –   To do two pleasurable activities each day –     To spend at least 15 minutes a day talking or playing with his children –     To do 20 minutes of physical exercise three times a week – To move towards employment |
| Treatment | Sharing the formulation with John was the first step. This helped him to understand why his thinking is so negative and how it related to his beliefs about illness and his perceived ability to cope.<br>It was important to liaise with his Diabetes Nurse. Sharing what he was doing in CBT helped him to develop a good relationship with her.<br>Behavioural approaches:<br>We used Behavioural Activation (BA) to reintroduce pleasurable activities, stabilise his daily routines (eating and sleeping) and to slowly introduce some more 'necessary' roles to increase his sense of achievement since finishing work.<br>'Little and often' was the motto we used, to make the 'all or nothing' rule more flexible and break his cycle of avoidance.<br>Cognitive approaches:<br>Attentional focus training was a big part of the cognitive work, to help him recognise and break the cycle of rumination. We used some grounding and mindfulness techniques to help him bring his attention back to the present moment.<br>NAT work included identifying his thoughts on a rumination diary.<br>Imagery work involved the development of a coping image. This included images of playing with his children and working again. This helped to modify his belief that he is weak.<br>Values-based approaches:<br>John was encouraged to view his Diabetes within the context of his whole life, across the domains of the values compass. He was able to identify other areas of his life that had become overshadowed by his diagnosis. This included studying, and he decided to enrol on a computer course to improve his IT skills. |
| Outcomes | After 10 sessions there was a significant improvement in John's symptoms of depression. He was more active in general, was spending more time doing activities with his family, had enquired by local driving jobs and was more positive about the future. |

Although we did not explicitly work on his beliefs about having Diabetes, he stated that he no longer sees it as a barrier to having a productive and satisfying life.
Relapse prevention was introduced early on in treatment and by the end he had developed a robust relapse prevention plan.

## Imagery re-scripting for depressive rumination with LTC

Imagery work has been recognised as a useful cognitive intervention for the psychological treatment of depression (Beck, 1979; Padesky, 2009). Despite the initial promotion of imagery for depression, it has become much more synonymous with treating the anxiety disorders, in particular trauma focused cognitive therapy (Ehlers & Clark, 2000) for PTSD (with the use of reliving). Imagery is also promoted in the Dugas and Robichaud (2007) model for GAD in the final module for increasing tolerance to distressing hypothetical worries through imaginal exposure. This is where a script is developed to encompass a troubling scenario, leaving it at a 'cliff hanger' for the person to habituate to the distress of not knowing how the scenario will end.

Imagery work for depression has tended to be overshadowed by the more dynamic approaches used in the anxiety disorders. This may be due to a belief that it is more useful for anxiety due to the clear and direct relationship of physiological arousal and avoidance (emotional and cognitive). Exposure work can see a dramatic shift in affect once the person habituates to the feared stimulus that they had been avoiding. With depression the biological symptoms can be misleading, as being physically sedentary does not mean that the brain is not physiologically aroused and causing mental distress. In fact, the content of depressive rumination is usually extremely negative, threatening and hopeless in nature, which leads to distress in the same way that anxiety does. The amygdala will fire when engaged in excessive rumination, and this will produce adrenaline and the unpleasant symptoms. The options to respond to this are fight, flight or freeze. Because depression produces so many biological symptoms that slows the body down – fatigue, poor sleep, lack of volition, motivation and loss of interest in people and things – then the person is much more likely to respond to the distress in the 'flight' (avoidance) or 'freeze' modes, keeping the person stuck in the distress. For this reason, it is essential that we use dynamic methods to break the cycle of rumination.

In a study to understand the role of information processing during depressive rumination, Brewin (2006) proposed the retrieval competition hypothesis. This is the idea that intrusive visual memories common in depressive rumination can be overridden by a more easily accessible positive image that is rehearsed. For example, if someone is preoccupied by negative traumatic memories of being physically abused by a parent, then an alternative image is scripted that reduces the negative impact of those memories, such as seeing the parent in shabby underwear or dressed as a baby with a dummy in their mouth. Once this image is repetitively inserted when the intrusive negative memory occurs, it becomes much easier to access and the emotional impact of the memory is supposed to be reduced. This is supported by Pearson, Brewin, Rhodes and McCarron (2015) who suggest that depression causes insufficient or weak positive future-focused imagery, so re-scripting can encourage prospective positive imagery (Blackwell et al., 2013) as well as re-shaping unpleasant memories of the past (Brewin et al., 2009).

Holmes, Crane, Fennell and Williams (2007), in their survey of people with depression, found that two-thirds of their sample reported experiencing visual imagery when ruminating on suicidal thoughts. Although a relatively small sample, others have also found high levels of imagery associated with depressive rumination (Pearson, Brewin, Rhodes & McCarron, 2008; Crane, Shah, Barnhofer & Holmes, 2012) suggesting that intrusive memories and rumination are mutually self-supporting. Moritz et al. (2014), reporting on the association of sensory properties of depressive thoughts, found that the most prevalent sensory experience was bodily, followed by auditory, with visual being the third most prevalent sensory experience. This was part of a large multi-centre study of on-line treatment for mild to moderate depression (Klein et al., 2013). These findings suggest that we should be using imagery techniques more often with our depressed patients. Arntz (2012) conducted a review of imagery work in CBT across different psychopathologies, showing the broad application and potential uses. Studies by Wheatley et al. (2007) and Brewin et al. (2009) show how imagery re-scripting can provide a stand-alone approach to treating depression without having to challenge or modify thoughts or beliefs. Whitaker, Brewin and Watson (2010) used imagery re-scripting with a patient who had been diagnosed with cancer, which helped him to develop a more nurturing image of being kind to himself. This supports the compassionate focused approach, where the creation of a self-compassionate alternative image is encouraged (Gilbert, 2005; Jacob et al., 2011). The overview by Wheatley and Hackmann (2011) of the use of imagery re-scripting for depression provides a comprehensive and accessible guide for practitioners to apply these techniques in patients with chronic depression. Referring back to the Klein et al. (2013) study, their recommendations regarding how imagery work could be integrated into psychological interventions for people with depression include; encouraging patients to vividly relive pleasant memories (Jacob et al., 2011), and develop other prospective positive imagery about the future (Blackwell et al., 2013; Williams, Blackwell, Mackenzie, Holmes & Andrews, 2013). This type of 'optimism imagery' fits well with patients with LTC and depression as their rumination will include uncertainty regarding how their health problems may change over time.

### Imagery work for intrusive memories and images relating to health fears

An early study of intrusive imagery in patients with health anxiety was conducted by Wells and Hackmann (1993). They identified three distinct themes of intrusive images, being focused on the self, death and illness, and were often linked to memories of adverse events. Muse, McManus, Hackman, Williams and Williams (2010) studied intrusive memories and images in severe health anxiety. The images tended to be future orientated, and were reliably categorised into four themes: 1) being told 'the bad news' that you have a serious/life threatening-illness (6.9%), 2) suffering from a serious or life-threatening illness (34.5%), 3) death and dying due to illness (22.4%) and 4) impact of own death or serious illness on loved ones (36.2%). In terms of imagery re-scripting, these categories can help us to form some alternative images that may compromise the emotional impact of the health-related intrusive images that plague people suffering with health anxiety and depression. Remember, that the combination of health anxiety and depression is particularly powerful in terms of the distress caused by excessive worry and rumination.

### Imagery work relating to self

These images are likely to involve images of being overwhelmed and not coping with a feared situation, or being in pain. Some alternatives to the image of the 'non-coping self' are:

- When the person gets the feared image, replace with an image of self with a super hero outfit on, looking strong, in control and powerful
- Use images of seeing yourself recover from an illness – such as leaving hospital looking proud and happy
- Images of helping others through a difficult and fearful time
- Images of the self as being bigger than the illness – have the illness written on a piece of paper in your hand and screw it into a ball and throw it away

Mooney and Padesky (2000) talk of patient creativity as an essential component in making meaningful changes, and how this requires a complete leap of faith by being open to imagine different possibilities in the future. This goes against the thinking biases common in depression and anxiety, that keep future focused thinking threat orientated and fixed. By encouraging patients to imagine a future where they are not victims to an illness but are coping, living with it, then the associated distress will be reduced. They sum this up eloquently: 'A focus on the future allows us to explore possibilities not yet imagined, to problem solve their application in our everyday life, and to experience a transformational shift in the paradigmatic ways we experience our world. Constructing possibilities, focusing on the new, fostering patient creativity and embracing ambiguity and doubt help clients integrate cognitive/analytical insights and emotional/experiential knowledge' (Mooney & Padesky, 2000, p. 160).

In terms of expanding the possibilities for the future, here is an exercise based on basic problem-solving strategies. It combines many of the theories presented in this section, to encourage more flexible and creative thinking rather than getting stuck on worst case scenario catastrophic thinking. It also embraces the threat-opportunity continuum idea, in order to expand the possibilities when the person imagines their future living with an LTC or MUS.

1    Imagine living with the LTC with the following possible outcomes:

    a    In pain but coping
    b    In pain and struggling
    c    Alone and coping
    d    Alone, depressed, and anxious
    e    Connected to people and values
    f    Helping others to live with the same problems

2    Imagine continuing to live with MUS:

    a    Mistrust of health care professionals
    b    Good relationships with health care professionals based on mutual trust
    c    Acceptance that doctors do not know everything
    d    Fighting to be taken seriously by friends and family
    e    Acceptance of own struggles without needing to convince others
    f    Life becoming more limited and lacking pleasure
    g    Opportunities to try new experiences that would not have been considered

Get the person to work through this list of scenarios and monitor how it makes them 'feel' when engaged in each one. Using the principle of retrieval competition hypothesis, help them to develop this image to insert when they find themselves engaged in excessive worry and rumination. Like problem-solving techniques, you want the person to be able to generate a creative selection of options, so they do not fall into an 'all or nothing' mind set when it comes to imagining their future living with an LTC or MUS. The imagery work described earlier (Wells & Hackman, 1993; Muse et al., 2010) led to the development and evaluation of Mindfulness based Cognitive Therapy (MBCT) interventions to treat intrusive images in severe health anxiety (McManus, Muse, Surwy, Hackman & Williams, 2015). This brings us full circle back to how the development of CBT has given rise to interventions that can all be adapted and targeted at reducing symptoms of depression when there is a co-morbid LTC

## Chapter summary

When depression is present in long-term conditions, this can be aided by low-intensity CBT, Beckian cognitive therapy, or recent approaches in the third wave tradition, including act and compassion focused therapy. This chapter has focused predominantly on the cognitive approach including a detailed account of Beck's CT for depression and special considerations when working with people with LTC. Imagery work, as a cognitive approach to working with depression with LTC is also outlined. Third wave approaches focusing on acceptance, diffusion, values and compassion are outlined and some techniques are described in detail in the next chapter.

# Chapter 6

# ACT and third wave approaches to depression in long-term conditions

Hayes (2004) is often cited as coining the phrase, 'waves' of therapy. There is a suggestion that a wave suggests a flow from one into the other, meaning that they represent development rather than distinct and exclusive approaches to treating mental distress. Clearly behaviourism and cognitive therapy have some distinct features as discussed in the previous chapter. A defining difference is in the use of traditional cognitive restructuring style techniques, which has been suggested, in dismantling studies, to be less effective or even unnecessary in comparison to behavioural techniques (Longmore & Worrell, 2007). This type of research has influenced the more recent resurgence of behavioural approaches in CBT. Acceptance and Commitment Therapy (ACT) has become popular more recently (Hayes, 2004) with an emphasis on acceptance of distressing states and commitment to changes in behaviour (Kennedy & Pearson, 2017). This approach emphasises acceptance as opposed to modification of beliefs, and a focus on values and compassion to encourage a more positive and meaningful approach to daily life. Arguably they incorporate both behavioural and cognitive elements as values are based on one's belief system. Some see ACT and compassion-focused therapy (Gilbert, 2010) as incorporating the best of both approaches, as they seek to help the person to act or behave in line with some principles, they not only value, but also serve to promote self-worth through acting in a more self-compassionate way. Interventions for all these approaches involve the use of role plays, metaphors and experiential exercises, some of which are presented later in this chapter.

Mindfulness plays a pivotal role in any third wave approach to CBT. Germer and Chan (2014) point out the difficulty in defining mindfulness due to its ineffable nature, though Kabat-Zinn's (1994, p. 4) definition is one of the most highly quoted: 'paying attention in a particular way: on purpose, in the present moment, and non-judgmentally.' It has long been recognised that worry and rumination focuses our attention away from the present moment, and prolongs the unpleasant feelings associated with unhappiness, fear, anger and other distressing emotions. We suggest that attentional focus training is an important element to any CBT intervention for LTC (and/or MUS). Pain and physical discomfort cause our attention to focus more on bodily sensations, which we then 'react' to by thinking and behaving in ways intended to reduce the pain. Of course, we know that this

DOI: 10.4324/9780367824433-9

increases the negative emotional response as a vicious cycle has been set up and maintained.

The studies suggest that ACT is effective for depression compared to no treatment, treatment-as-usual, or placebo conditions. It is less clear how ACT compares to CBT due to the number of trials and tendency for small sample sizes in existing studies, but results suggest it is likely at least equally effective for depression (Twohig & Levin, 2017). A 2016 analysis of 18 studies of ACT in Chronic disease and LTC reported on 18 studies: eight were randomised controlled trials (RCTs), four used pre–post designs, and six were case studies. A broad range of applications was observed (e.g. improving quality of life and symptom control, reducing distress) across many diseases/conditions (e.g. HIV, cancer, epilepsy). However, study quality was low, and many interventions were of low intensity. The small number of RCTs per application and lower study quality emphasise that ACT is not yet a well-established intervention for chronic disease/long-term conditions (Graham, Gouick, Krahe & Gillanders, 2016)

Some of the differences and similarities between CBT and ACT have been described earlier. Acceptance and commitment therapy focuses on flexibility:

- Acceptance (that the patient works on trying to except the reality of his pain or physical condition, not wanting it or liking it, and acknowledging that battling with it has more disadvantages and advantages)
- Present moment awareness (the patient is fully in touch with what is happening in the moment good or bad, this means not dwelling in worry or rumination)
- Defusion (this means that the patient is defused with his experiences, for example seeing his negative thoughts as separate from himself)
- Self as a context (experiencing one's life story is something that is happening now, and stepping away from the narrative of oneself as a cancer sufferer or an ill person)
- Committed action (the person takes steps he has made a commitment to, towards what is important for him)
- Values (the person is very engaged in what is profoundly important in his life)

## Practical exercises for depression and LTC using third wave approaches

The exercises presented in this section are effective for treating depression with or without a long-term condition. However, each exercise has some additional suggestions in terms of how to adapt them to focus specifically on the themes and cognitions that may be implicated when there is a co-morbid LTC. There are three different categories of exercises we will present. The first section looks at attentional focus strategies. The second considers values, and the concluding section presents theory and practical exercises relating to imagery work.

## *Attentional focus training exercises*

### *The watering can*

This is an experiential exercise that we have found helpful in depression to show the emotional impact of rumination and worry, and we will describe it in detail.

### *Use of metaphor*

Using the metaphor of water to represent our attention, draw a watering can and state that the full can is 100% of our attention in any given moment. Then draw three plants that need water – the PAST, PRESENT and FUTURE. All start the same size. Ask the patient to estimate how much water each plant is currently receiving. Emphasise that the past refers to time spent in RUMINATION, and the future is time spent actively engaged in WORRY. State that it is possible to do tasks and have a conversation in the PRESENT but that the whirring of worry and rumination may still be drawing their attention inwards. So, you should now

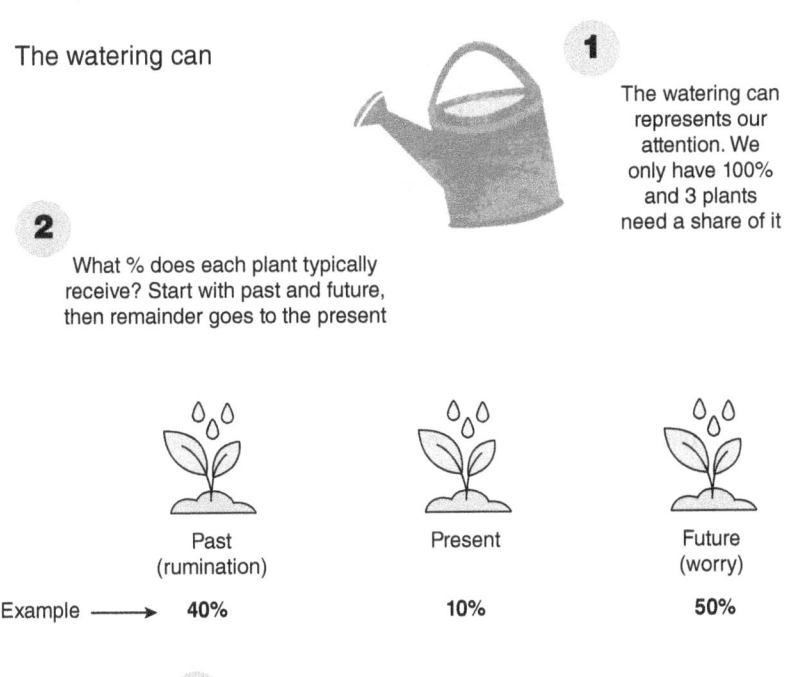

Figure 6.1 Watering can

have percentages assigned to each plant. Give the patient a couple of moments to reflect on this, then state that you are going to do something with this information.

### Live experiment phase

On the other side of the paper draw two equal graphs, with Emotion on the X axis and Time on the Y axis. Graph one will be titled PAST or RUMINATION and Graph two will be titled FUTURE or WORRY. Underneath the graph there will be a key with the main negative emotions such as SAD, FEAR, GUILT, ANGER. Include any other relevant ones that fit your client's problem such as DISGUST in an OCD obsessive presentation where the person may engage in excessive obsessive rumination. Give each emotion a colour code.

### Condition 1

Ask person to close their eyes and actively ruminate. Prompt them by saying something like 'draw to mind something that has already happened that you think about a lot and find hard to let go of' or 'draw to mind a thought or memory that you find you get stuck on'. Ask them to describe the thought then use some Socratic Questioning to get them to articulate the movement of the thought. Examples are:

'and where does that take your thinking now?'
'and what is the worst thing about that thought?'
'and what does that thought make you conclude about yourself?'

After about 2–3 minutes, ask them to open their eyes. Immediately move onto the next step while they are still feeling the emotional impact of the exercise. Ask them to plot on the graph which emotions they FELT whilst ruminating (not whilst in the situations recounted). It is likely that they felt more than one. For example, recounting an argument with a partner may make them feel sad, guilty and angry at different points of the rumination and to different degrees. I always emphasise that this is not an exact science (the graphical representation of the feelings), but that it provides an opportunity to recognise the emotional impact that rumination has, even when only engaged in for 2–3 minutes.

### Condition 2

Now repeat the process described in Condition 1 using a FUTURE focus, asking them to draw to mind something that hasn't happened yet (and may never happen) that they are worried about. You say something like 'draw to mind a what if'. It makes sense to get them to worry about the future in terms of the worries related to having an LTC or MUS. The clinician should not be afraid of causing distress as the aim of this exercise is to help them to learn how emotionally distressing it is when their attention is focused on their condition and the associated worries and rumination.

**4** Get the person to actively ruminate for a couple of minutes with eyes closed, then rate emotions they felt. Repeat with worry.

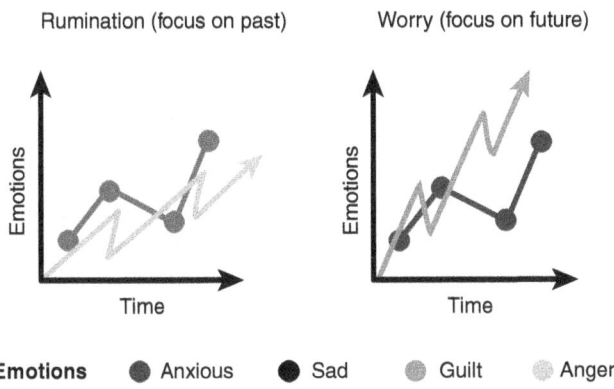

**5** Finish the exercise with a mindful meditation to contrast the emotional distress when worrying and rumination to being in the present moment

*Figure 6.2* Rumination graph

Some prompts include:

'what if your symptoms get worse? Then. . . .'
'what if I never know what is wrong with me? What would be the worst thing about that?
'what if I have to take medication for the rest of my life? That would mean. . .'

After 2–3 minutes ask them to open their eyes and immediately plot the graph. It is important that they make the connection between the worry and the intense feelings this causes.

### Bringing attention back to the present moment

At this point you emphasise how important it is that we can shift attention back to the present moment in order to break the cycle of rumination and worry. You can refer to the watering can and plants, reiterating that the PRESENT plant is very dry and needs more of the water from the watering can. Ask the person how they think we can bring our attention back to the present moment. Often, they are unsure. Here are some ways of setting the stage for some mindfulness type exercise. We say that when the brain is in distress (refer to diagram and limbic system) this causes the unpleasant symptoms, and when this occurs, we go onto auto-pilot and sensory information is 'dumbed down.' Therefore, our heads feel so FULL. Again, use the water analogy. I (Helen) want to override this by ramping up the sensory information we pay attention to. At this point I do a guided mindful meditation with the person. Here are some suggestions:

- Prior to the meditation I offer a concentrated essential oil, such as lavender or rose, and if they like the smell I ask them to put a little on their hand and inhale deeply.
- I ask them to close their eyes and start the meditation by taking three deeper breaths than normal, focusing on the sensations of the breath
- I do a brief body scan starting with the feet
- I state how difficult this can be and use a METAPHOR for thoughts and thinking such as leaves on a tree than fall into a river and float away
- Reiterate that there is no such thing as 'doing it wrong', it just takes practice
- Emphasise that attention is being pulled back to the trees and river, but that they can come back to the breath and their feet
- Move the body scan up their body to the parts connected to the chair they are sitting in, encouraging a more focused attention on how it feels
- Add other mindful techniques using the other senses such as mindful listening – tuning into the sounds around them
- When attention is pulled back to the thoughts, they can gently nudge it back to their senses
- End with some deeper breaths and gently return to the room

On opening their eyes, the therapist asks them to describe how the experience was for them. Often, but not always, they will describe feeling calmer than the first two conditions where they were actively ruminating or worrying. This is the experiential learning you are trying to achieve. At this point you want them to commit to trying this practice between sessions. I show them some examples of free apps they can use, and encourage them to download them straight away. This minimises the opportunity for avoidance.

Emphasise that this practice should be used not only when already distressed, in a grounding manner, but also at other times in order to prevent build-up of emotional distress through excessive worry and rumination. Again, the metaphor of the watering can helps to reinforce the benefit of not letting your head get so full that it overflows. Watering the PRESENT plant will keep them grounded for longer. Like any exercise it will take practice.

Cautionary notes regarding mindfulness meditation and LTC or MUS

Be aware that sometimes when people have physical health conditions, or MUS, doing a meditation such as that described earlier, can intensify their symptoms, which in turn can cause emotional distress. Some patients describe feeling overwhelmed and unable to focus attention away from the source of their physical sensations or symptoms. As with all CBT interventions and education, reiterate the value of the experiential learning and how they can reflect on this, rather than dismiss it as unsuitable or a failure. Some of the common issues that lead to distress in these circumstances and how they can be addressed are presented in Table 6.1.

*Table 6.1* Cautions around mindfulness

| Cause of distressing reaction | Potential reasons and resolutions |
| --- | --- |
| Person becomes distressed and reports that they are feeling extremely anxious | They may be focusing on these physical sensations associated with anxiety such as heart rate. |
| | Demonstrate how focusing attention on one area of the body will intensify the sensations, and practice moving attention away from that one area using the other senses of moving the body scan to other areas of the body, or focusing on breath or sounds. |
| | Do this quickly so that they are not reluctant to try again, as they are unlikely to do it by themselves after the session |
| Person reports that that were unable to move their attention away from the thoughts, or kept slipping back to the rumination and worry | Explain that this is normal when you first start mindful meditation to be very distractable. |
| | Explain the difference between this and other types of meditation in terms of the aims. It is important that they do not hold beliefs about meditation in general that may be interfering with their experience of it during this exercise. For example, that they need to clear their mind completely to achieve the 'clean slate.' |
| | You can also try using an alternative metaphor for thoughts and thinking, such as the train coming through the station and you do not want to be focusing too much attention looking back or forward or jumping on the train as it goes round and round. |
| Person reports feeling physically uncomfortable | Meditation that takes place whilst sitting down can cause discomfort, especially to those who may have muscular-skeletal or other physical symptoms and chronic pain. Merely sitting in a chair in one position can cause discomfort and this will override any attentional focus on the meditation guidance. |
| | Try mindful movement or other mindfulness activity that will still encourage the shifting of attention back to the present moment. Some ideas are presented as follows. |

## Alternatives to mindful meditation in chairs during the session

If meditation is not desired, or considered unsuitable for any of the reasons described earlier, then immediately after the active rumination and worry conditions the therapist can try one of the following activities:

- Use mindful movement, by guiding the person to focus on how it feels to be moving around the room, perhaps saying 'You can still focus attention on the other senses but you won't be mixed in position in a chair. Take it outside and really ramp up the sensory information around you'.
- Ask the person to do 5–10 minutes of mindful colouring straight after the active rumination and worry conditions. Ask them to focus on the colours and patterns, and check in with their emotional experience whilst doing this
- Do a puzzle with the person such as Jenga or a jigsaw

The important part of this exercise is the experiential learning, so be sure to help the person focus on how they are feeling at the end of the whole exercise and get immediate feedback. Ensure they record their feedback on the sheet so they capture this important learning. At this point I (HM), direct them to some free apps that provide brief mindful meditations. Ideally ask them to download at least one at the end of the session. I have some on my phone and always open one to show them as I think it is more likely they will engage with them if they have seen one.

Homework tasks can include:

- Practicing the mindful meditations using the app
- Increase awareness of using their senses by setting mundane daily tasks to be approached mindfully, such as cleaning teeth or eating a snack
- Setting a 10-minute mindful walk as a homework task is not only good for attentional focus training, it can increase overall activity and encourage them to get out of the house. This is vital for breaking the cycle of rumination and avoidance in depression. You may need to adapt in LTC where mobility is compromised.

## Attention and pain

When pain is a daily experience for someone with LTC and MUS, it can become the focus of their attention throughout the day. Several safety and avoidance behaviours are likely to ensue and this sets up a vicious cycle based on the threat-drive mechanism – where pain is viewed to be the threat and the person will drive to eliminate it through the safety and avoidance behaviours. Pain becomes something to try and control, which is extremely difficult if not impossible, so the fight continues.

With pain, from an ACT and compassion-focused perspective, the aim is to help the person to accept that the pain is there, and reduce the safety and avoidance behaviours that feed into the distress created by having a high focus of attention on pain. Here is another exercise that we have found useful:

*Physicalising pain exercise:* this exercise can be presented as a mindful meditation, beginning by getting the person to get into a comfortable position and begin with some slow breaths. With eyes closed, ask the person to imagine all their pain moving to one area such as their stomach. Now ask them to put their hands on their stomach and imagine pulling the pain out and holding it in front of them. Encourage them to examine the pain, describing how it looks and feels in their hands. Be creative here and let the person explore the idea of being able to interact with the pain. If it could talk what would they say to it and what might the pain say to them?

*Drawing pain:* like the physicalising pain exercise, you can ask the person to draw themselves and mark their pain on the drawing. Encourage the exploration of other areas of their body and enhance these, so that pain can be placed in perspective. This is another way of helping to distance from the overshadowing effect that pain has on attention.

*Band of light;* this is a mindfulness meditation technique, not exclusively used for the management of pain. In this exercise ask the person to close their eyes and imagine a band of light starting at either their head moving down their body, or from their feet up. Focus on the light for a few moments and let it enter the body and fill it up. Encourage curiosity in terms of how this light may soothe and calm the mind and body. Reference to pain may or may not be made, as the light may perform different functions to the person in this meditation. Issues can be explored afterwards, such as what impact this had on the experience of their pain before, during and after the meditation.

*Attentional focus 'then and now' – Photo review exercise:* attentional focus is affected when we look back at old photos. Often, we will focus on ourselves and quickly conclude about whether the photo evokes positive or negative feelings. For example, a photo taken 10 years ago on a holiday that the patient really enjoyed may evoke happiness at the memory of the holiday, whilst simultaneously or very quickly changing to a negative feeling fuelled by thoughts of how much they have changed physically – 'I look so young and slim on there, but look at me now. I was really healthy then'. These judgements will impact on mood, and may be even more pronounced in someone who has an LTC or MUS which limits activities they can currently engage in. So, for this person, looking at the holiday photo from 10 years ago may cause them to ruminate on losses – to physical health, and other activities or career opportunities. We really want the person to gain a broader perspective than the dichotomous – before and after (physical health problems) all or nothing style of thinking that is implicated in depression. Despite a range of life circumstances that may have been challenging in the person's past, there will be a tendency to believe that 'before' was always better than now – due to the perceived losses.

*Broadening perspective when looking at old photos:* rather than making a snap judgement on a photo, we want the person to engage in a broader analysis of their

*Table 6.2* Photo review

| Positive things from the photo I still value | Things that are better in my life now |
| --- | --- |
| I might look older now and not as slim but I still look good for my age | During that time, I was unhappy at work, but changed careers and am much happier now |
| I can still go on nice holidays | We paid for that holiday on my credit card and it took a year to pay it off, which was stressful |
| I still enjoy time with my wife and children | The children have grown up and we have more time as a couple and less monthly expenses |

life at that time in order to recognise both what they can still do that they did then, and to consider some of the things that may be better now than at the time of the photo, for example 'it was a lovely holiday, but that was the time I was unhappy at work and life was really difficult until I changed jobs'.

Table 6.2 presents some examples of questions and issues you can explore when the person examines the old photo.

By interrogating the photo for more information, the perspective is expanding from the rose-coloured lens which leads to the conclusion that life was always better before 'I got Diabetes', or 'coronary heart disease'. So, ask the person to collect examples of photos over the past few years and repeat this exercise for each one. In particular, use a recent photo and spend time exploring the range of thoughts that go through the person's mind when they look at themselves in the here-and-now. Use Socratic questioning to link beliefs at each level to their formulation, and explore meanings of these judgements. For example, if they say 'I look old and tired,' you can ask 'other than focusing of those factors, what else can you say about yourself at this time?,' or 'how do you think your wife/children/ best friend would answer that question?'

## Values-based exercises

Another category of exercises, commonly used within an ACT approach, involve the exploration of values (Kennedy & Pearson, 2017). We have considered how acceptance involves paying attention to current experience, now we turn our attention to how commitment to changes can be encouraged.

*Values compass:* a good exercise to help gain perspective is the values compass. This incorporates the ideas from ACT, the importance to remaining true to your personal values, especially during times of adversity and challenge. At these times, when life is more difficult and our mood is low it is easy to lose sight of our personal philosophy of life. As already stated, when depressed our thinking is negative and we develop biases in how we process information. One or two areas of our life can have an overshadowing effect on the other aspects of. This is common when we are suffering with a physical health condition. This can become our primary focus of attention from the moment we wake up and start our day. For the values compass, draw a compass and place different important domains of your life around the points of the compass.

These are some of the domains: Family, Education, Work/occupation, Health Leisure, Partnership/intimacy, spirituality, Community activity and integration, Friendships, Parenting, Aspirations and goals. For each of the domains, ask the person to reflect on what is important to them and write this down under the heading. This can be done on flash cards or post-it notes to show how flexible and moveable they are, rather than being rigid and fixed. Lay them out and ask the person to point the compass to the values that are currently dominating their lives, and discuss the impact of this on the other areas. For example, if someone has an LTC or MUS that has meant they can no longer do the career or occupation they are highly skilled in and love, PHYSICAL HEALTH and WORK are likely to overshadow the other areas. This means that rumination and worry about health and work are likely to dominate their lives and prevent connection to their other values. This exercise can be adapted in many ways and is enhanced by Socratic Questioning to maximise the potential for guided discovery. Helping people to recognise there is untapped potential in other areas of their lives that they are not currently paying attention to can develop sufficient shift in thinking and behaviour to motivate positive change.

## Values compass

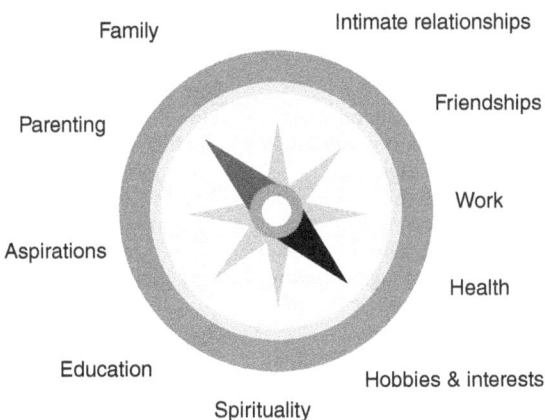

**NB.)** *This list is not exhaustive and can be developed collaboratively*

*Figure 6.3* Values compass

### Integrating values into everyday life

Once values have been identified and brought into conscious awareness, we need to encourage the person to monitor when they are and are not adhering to these values. Kennedy and Pearson (2017) provide an example of how people can become more aware of whether they are orientating to their values in these areas by reflecting on their behaviours during the past week that supported the values, and the behaviours that did not. We suggest that this exercise can be extended to include new goals based on this information for the week ahead. Table 6.3 is adapted from Kennedy and Pearson (2017, p. 75).

*Table 6.3* Monitoring and planning to integrate values

| My values | My Actions last week | | Small steps towards my values this week |
| --- | --- | --- | --- |
| <u>Relationships</u><br>Being understanding<br>Being forgiving<br>Being approachable<br>Spending time together | In line:<br>Didn't hang onto resentment when husband upset me<br>Helped son with homework even when I was tired | Out of line:<br>Snapped at my daughter when she didn't agree with me<br>Didn't interact with family at the weekend. Spent more time alone in bed. | Have mealtimes with family at weekend even if tired or in pain<br>Try and listen and accept others' views without reacting<br>Forgive self when I have snapped or lost control |
| <u>How I occupy my day</u><br>Using my skills at work<br>Trying my best | In line:<br>Finished project at work and was pleased with it | Out of line:<br>Rushed through the accounts and made some errors | Pace self and prioritise tasks at work |
| <u>Leisure/growth</u><br>Learning new skills<br>Maintaining my hobbies<br>Meeting new people | In line:<br>Introduced myself to the new neighbour<br>Sorted the computer problem without asking someone to do it for me | Out of line:<br>Didn't go to ballet as I was too tired<br>Made an excuse when friend asked me to go out | Try and go to ballet this week<br>Look for other dance classes that might start at a more convenient time |
| <u>Health</u><br>Eat healthily<br>Exercise<br>Take my medication<br>Ask for help when needed<br>Regular sleep pattern | In line:<br>Had a small walk 4 days of the week<br>Ordered my repeat prescription<br>Told husband I couldn't do shopping due to pain | Out of line:<br>Skipped meals and overate most evenings<br>Stayed up on laptop until after 2 am most nights watching Netflix | Don't use laptop in bed. Play calming music or meditate.<br>Draw up a meal plan and include family |

This template can be used to help the person identify gaps in their values-based behaviours, and target these as daily or weekly goals. It is important that the goals are set as very small steps in order to make them realistic and achievable, particularly when pain and fatigue are daily challenges. Rather than highlighting deficits, we want the person to accept that values, like any other behaviours, do not function in an all-or-nothing manner. We want to encourage a gentle nudge towards behaviours that are more consistent with their values rather than judging these as 'good' or 'bad.' The rationale for this is to make their thinking and behaviours more flexible in order to alleviate some of the symptoms of depression and/or anxiety caused when their behaviours are out of line with what they value.

## Chapter Summary

This chapter has presented a selection of methods to support an ACT approach to depression with LTC: these include the use of metaphor, imagination and creativity. The emphasis is on attentional focus and values.

Chapter 7

# Skills in working with anxiety disorders in long-term conditions

## Health anxiety

As we consider health anxiety here, we can look initially at a generic model and we can also consider how it manifests itself in long-term conditions: the CBT formulation of health anxiety, (which is sometimes called hypochondriasis, or illness anxiety disorder), has some features in common with the CBT formulation of panic disorder. Patients with health anxiety dwell on physical symptoms and worry excessively about their health. The CBT model of health anxiety (Salkovskis, 1989) specifies it as a condition where the health anxious individual develops a preoccupation that he has, or will develop, a serious, usually fatal, disease. This preoccupation is based on catastrophic misinterpretations of bodily sensations, where the threat and danger are future orientated (e.g. 'I am going to die of cancer soon'). This future orientation can be contrasted with the CBT model of panic disorder, where there is also a catastrophic misinterpretation of bodily sensations but the threat and danger are imminent (e.g. 'I am going to have a heart attack now').

Examples of misinterpretations in health anxiety are:

- 'Headache means brain tumour'
- 'Lump means cancer'
- 'Muscle cramps means multiple sclerosis'
- 'Diarrhoea/stomach pains means bowel cancer'
- 'Aching jaw means bone cancer'
- 'Irregular heartbeat means heart disease'
- 'Changes to skin colour means skin cancer'

Imagery is important in health anxiety and the content includes how the person may die (a long, slow death, with much pain and suffering), or what will happen after death (abandoned and alone in a cold dark grave), or how the lives of loved ones will be once the person is dead (partner will meet someone else, and the deceased will be quickly forgotten by their partner and children). Such imagery is often linked to rules for living and core beliefs. For an excellent clinical discussion of the role of imagery in the maintenance of health anxiety, see Wells and

DOI: 10.4324/9780367824433-10

Hackmann (1993). Typical themes for rules for living and core beliefs in health anxiety include control, and perceived dangerousness, for example core beliefs, 'I am vulnerable', 'I am weak', 'the world is dangerous', 'I am vulnerable to ill health'; the rule is 'If I'm not in control then something bad will happen'. Intolerance of uncertainty is prominent for example 'The future is uncertain, this is threatening and I can't accept this.'

As in panic disorder, benign bodily sensations are perceived as threatening or dangerous and this raises anxiety levels. These symptoms of anxiety are then taken as further evidence of ill health and bodily sensations are intensified, which focuses attention on symptoms, and increases a preoccupation with illness. Information processing biases, often threat cue detection, leads the sufferer to scan their bodies for symptoms of ill health, and this is a key maintenance factor. This preoccupation with signs of ill health leads to reassurance seeking from medical sources, which may include frequent visits to the General Practitioner, attendance at Accident and Emergency, logging on to the internet, or reading relevant literature or websites to check out the meaning of symptoms, and asking a trusted person for reassurance regarding symptoms. Safety behaviours are also important factors in the maintenance of health anxiety, and examples include behaviours such as pulse checking, prodding relevant parts of the body to check for signs of abnormality (e.g. lumps), and repeatedly mechanically moving a part of the body where pain is experienced, in order to check out if it has lessened or worsened.

Typical activating events in health anxiety would be unusual, persistent, or intense bodily sensations such as headaches, dizziness, palpitations, breathlessness, pains and discomforts. External activating events may also include being exposed to health information, or the illness or death of a family member. As mentioned, at the level of information processing, the patient will excessively attend to potentially threatening bodily sensations, and these may be amplified. Worry and rumination on future and past illness experiences of themselves or others is prominent. Intolerance of uncertainty is prominent.

Health anxiety often occurs co-morbidly with generalised anxiety disorder and depression. Most people who present with the problem recognise they have always worried about their health, and often there is a family history of such concerns. In terms of CBT treatment, a standard intervention is around 10–15 sessions but it is a difficult problem to treat, as engagement takes time, and the excessive need for reassurance seeking, if not managed effectively, will seriously undermine treatment. Often patients who present with health anxiety are viewed as problematic particularly in relation to requests for medical investigations. Possible underlying issues of dependency can make the problem more complex to treat. However, a systematic review and meta-analysis (Cooper, Gregory, Walker, Lambe & Salkovskis, 2017) provides support for the hypothesis that CBT is an effective intervention for health anxiety when compared with a variety of control conditions, for example treatment-as-usual, waiting list, medication and other psychological therapies.

Tyrer et al. (2011) investigated the prevalence of health anxiety in general (hospital) medical clinics (the 'CHAMP study') and found a high incidence: of 43,205 patients attending the clinics 28,991 (67.1%) were assessed and of these, after exclusion of ineligible patients 5,747 (19.8%) had significant health anxiety. The prevalence levels varied by clinic with neurology (24.7%), having the highest prevalence, followed by respiratory medicine (20.9%), gastroenterology (19.5%), cardiology (19.1%) and endocrinology (17.5%). The study reports that the type of people who attend the clinic and the fact that it was done by questionnaire, may affect the outcomes. Tyrer et al. (2014), in a later study, compared 'treatment as usual' to health anxiety CBT, and found that patients had sustained systematic improvement to their anxiety symptoms from CBT over two years, but there was no economic benefit. A further study showed no decline in improvement at five years (Tyrer et al., 2017). CBT did not lead to greater secondary improvements in 'social functioning or quality of life', compared to TAU. This treatment was delivered by graduate workers, assistant psychologists and general nurses, the latter group interestingly proving to be the most effective therapists.

Health anxiety skills:

- assessment is broadly the same as any anxiety disorder, but ensure all reassurance seeking is understood
- Help engage the patient with a credible formulation. So, ensure patient understands that safety behaviours and reassurance are counterproductive.
- Emphasise that we would not wish the patient to miss early signs of an illness if one was there
- Help the patient to give up reassurance at an early stage
- Be skilful in helping the patient to gradually drop Safety Behaviours like bodily checking
- Be skilful in negotiating when it is reasonable for the patient to consult the GP.

Here is a session-by-session guide to treatment based on standard approaches (Salkovskis & Warwick, 1986; Tyrer, 2013).

1  *Assess* presenting problem. Measure problem using *Health anxiety inventory* (Salkovskis, Rimes & Warwick, 2002)
2  Finish assessment. Develop *formulation* collaboratively (could use Salkovskis formulation, vicious flower) and agree treatment plan. Explain the theory A 'That you have cancer', and theory B 'that you're worried about having cancer', concept. Give out handout or suggest book for example 'Overcoming health anxiety' by Veale and Willson (2009). Get the patient to keep a *diary of events, symptoms and anxiety levels* (health anxiety thought record, first three columns)
3  Do *Problem and Targets*. Review their diary. Use a *pie chart* (draw on paper) to help the patient evaluate the different causes of a symptom. (Get them to

list all the causes of a symptom, and how likely each cause is as a percentage). Use the *inverted pyramid* (drawing it on paper) to help them evaluate how likely a given symptom will be dangerous or fatal. Set them homework of using a pie chart and inverted pyramid every time they have a symptom, and ask them to bring it in next session. (A workable alternative to this would be the use of the diary already used, but to complete the remaining columns of the diary, challenging the health anxious thoughts).

4   Review their use of the pie chart and inverted pyramid (or diary). These should help the patient to consider that they are catastrophising about their health.

5   Re-explain the concept of *safety seeking behaviours (SBs)*, including body checking and monitoring, reassurance seeking (including verbal reassurance and requests for medical investigations), and 'poking and prodding', emphasising why they are unhelpful (explaining this is because they increase preoccupation, stop healthy learning, and may make the symptoms worse). Ask them to evaluate the effect of checking and other SBs, doing them versus not doing them (they could try a week each), measuring anxiety, health preoccupation, and functioning in each condition. Over time we would expect to find that SBs worsen these scores, though they may initially decrease them. (If the patient already recognises the negative effect of SBs, it is reasonable to go to next step)

6   Review the effect of SBs by reviewing the diary. Set behavioural experiments to stop SBs. Agree behavioural experiments to tackle avoidance, for example of going to the doctors, or being with sick people

7   Review reduction of SBs and ongoing homework as appropriate

8   Review reduction of SBs and ongoing homework as appropriate. Help patient to address thinking processes like *worry* if this is a problem. Address positive beliefs about worry if present. Add evidence into the theory A and theory B sheet.

9   Help patients work with *core beliefs and rules* for living, if appropriate: using changing the rules sheet and continuum. Give out *relapse prevention* activity sheet.

10  Review homework with core beliefs and rules for living. Go over Relapse prevention activity sheet. Administer health anxiety scale again, and review Problems and targets.

11  Optional: *Consider other techniques commonly used* 1) problem solving, 2) Living a healthy lifestyle, 3) imagery re-scripting of a key incident that is currently present as a distressing image, for example, of a relative getting cancer, 4) exposure to their worst fears, for example, of being dead, being very ill, being dependent. This could be done as a pure exposure exercise, or to explore coping strategies.

12  As per 12

13  Follow-up session: review relapse prevention plan and update of necessary. Do measurement using *Health anxiety scale*, and review Problems and Goals.

14  Further follow-up: review relapse prevention plan and update of necessary. Do measurement using *Health anxiety scale*, and review Problems and
targets.

### Reassurance seeking as a problem

Re-assurance can be a big problem here, and the cognitions associated with this
are, 'I won't be able to stand it if I can't be sure what's wrong with me', or 'I've
got something seriously wrong with me', 'I compare my symptoms to what they
were yesterday by poking and prodding my body just to make sure they are the
same'. The patient's behaviour may be: mentally scanning their body to try to
identify symptoms and to make a comparison to how they have been previously;
to go on the Internet, using the search term around what they are worried about,
and then comparing the information on the Internet with their impression of their
symptoms; go to the doctor and describing symptoms they are worried about on a
very regular basis. We would have a discussion with the patient about the negative
effects of these behaviours, which are that they will be giving contradictory information, which will increase their anxiety; that if they poke and prod their body,
(because they are not medically qualified), they will not be able to properly interpret the findings. Experiments here will be to reduce and stop the safety and reassurance behaviour, and make a number of observations, possibly on a 0–100%
scale: this will be their level of anxiety, the ability to focus on normal day-to-day
tasks, the severity of the symptoms that they are worried about, and the actual
instance of diagnosed ill health. We would ask her to have one week in which
the reassurance and safety behaviours are continued, and then one week where
they are stopped. It is not easy for the patient to stop the safety behaviours and
this may have to be done in a gradual way. The advantage of doing this weekly
comparison, is that a direct comparison can be made between the effects of using
and not using reassurance. One would expect that the scores would be overall
better when the reassurance is not used. In the spirit of behavioural experiments,
if certain outcomes are not as expected, then this can be explored Socratically: it
may be difficult, for example, for the person to make a judgement as to whether
they develop a serious illness after a trial of a few experiments. Another discovery
behavioural experiment will be associated with the cognition 'I have a physical
illness;' the patient can be asked to read a medical journal about the condition or
to obtain objective medical information.

### What are the challenges of treating heath anxiety?

There can be a big problem in getting the patient alongside with the formulation, this may be because they think that if they have a course of CBT, then their
medical problems will be ignored, or they may think that they may be allowing a
problem like cancer to get worse, while they have psychological treatment. The
best way is to explore whether their previous ways of coping with their problems

have worked and ask whether they are willing to give another approach a try. This consent may hinge on whether they have enough confidence that they problem is anxiety based: this consideration can be strengthened if preliminary treatment brings about some improvements, so early gains are something that should be aspired to. Likewise putting data in the Theory A and Theory B sheet, should help this. Another problem can be that patients, if they do not have presenting symptoms, can present as quite well, and ready for discharge, whereas in fact the health anxiety system is not being activated at this moment, this is a kind of yo-yo effect. So, the therapist needs to engage the affect to ensure that the CBT sills are being used effectively.

### What to do differently if the person has a medical disorder/long-term condition?

If the patient has an actual medical health problem (current or long-term), this makes things more complicated. Nevertheless, Cooper's et al. (2017) study showed that the effects of CBT outcome were not diminished by including people who had an actual medical condition. So, this meta-analysis provides evidence that realistic automatic thoughts are not a treatment barrier, and so this medically ill group should be offered CBT treatment for their HA. In this medically ill group, the patient needs to strike a balance between vigilance towards symptoms, and not fuelling health anxiety due to preoccupation: a useful question is 'what do your medical health experts say about this symptom?' It is also important to remind the person that if they are anxious, they will always 'catastrophise'. Sometimes the patient develops new symptoms whilst one is treating them, and there is a question as to how to react, especially if the person has a medical disorder. What we would do, and encourage the patient to do, is to consider whether the symptoms are: 1) new, 2) severe and 3) persistent. So, if they meet all or some of this criterion, it may be wise to get them evaluated by the GP, but not if they do not significantly meet this criterion. As part of treatment, we would get the patient to adopt this approach to evaluating new symptoms, as we believe this is a reasonable approach, and may be applicable with Covid issues.

A typical scenario here is that a person does have a diagnosis of cancer or heart disease or diabetes, but also has a set of symptoms that have not been clearly linked to the original diagnosis. This situation can leave the patient anxious about the cause of the new symptoms. One can consider in therapy whether the symptoms seem more like a manifestation of anxiety or can be more credibly explained by the underlying disease process, this can be helped by the theory A theory B process. There are some great specific examples of CBT procedures in the second part of Helen Tyrer's book: the main advice she gives is that health anxiety is common amongst the medically ill, a diary is helpful to look at the triggers for the symptoms, patients should be given credible explanations for their symptoms in terms of muscle tension or hyperventilation in anxiety causing increased carbon dioxide, causing tingling and light headedness. Earlier medical communications that patients may have misunderstood need to be clarified, and one should use the standard CBT techniques for health anxiety.

Clinical example: a year before being seen, Jackie (Philip's patient) had her breast partly removed because of cancer. At the time of CBT assessment, she described her main problem as being frightened that the cancer was going to re-occur. This is triggered by memories of the cancer, and some physical/pain symptoms that she experiences. The specific worries that she has are 'if the cancer re-occurs, I will definitely die', and 'my family would be left behind.' When she gets these thoughts, she becomes very anxious, with a feeling of tension, dry mouth, breathlessness, and heart racing. She becomes very vigilant to her body and she engages in a number of reassurance-type strategies, the main one being excessively attending her GP and breast care nurse. She also does sometimes over check her breast, but at other times she prefers to avoid checking. She can look at her scar, but if she notices any changes she will start thinking 'is this lumpy?', 'is it different from how it was?', and she may examine her breast as much as three to four times weekly. Onset of the problem was three months prior, she developed severe pain in the breast, this had led to distress from the pain, reassurance seeking about relapse (even although she has been told that she has not relapsed). She says she feels depressed and has physical symptoms of tiredness. She feels ashamed she is not coping, thinking that's she's 'weak.' However, in general she is trying to get on with her life normally by swimming, looking after her grandchildren, going to her caravan, and this is going fairly-well. She describes her personality as putting other people first, not to show any anxiety, to but a brave face on. She sometimes thinks 'it's weak if I talk about my illness,'. This attitude can lead to traits of suppressing her feelings, and not always asking for support from her friends and family. On the other hand, her personality is quite positive and humorous. Her self-esteem and confidence were low as a child, particularly because of dyslexia, but are reasonable now.

I (PK) tried to work with Jackie to decide what the main problem was, and we agreed that this was essentially a health anxiety problem, because although she has had cancer there is no evidence that this is currently active. We developed a formulation looking at the role of catastrophic thinking, excessive checking and reassurance seeking: we thought that the catastrophic thinking raised her anxiety levels and these physiological symptoms could be misinterpreted, the ensuing anxiety would lead to a shift in attention towards the symptoms which will magnify them. The planning of SBs leads to a sense that there is something dangerous that needs to be protected against, and the execution of the SBs stops Jackie learning that she would be safe without doing them, this also applied to reassurance seeking. We acknowledged that she found it difficult to express her feelings and accept help, because of her rule for living.

The treatment approach here consisted of measuring the level of health anxiety using the health anxiety inventory, using theory a and theory b. Because she was getting a lot of pain this was evidence that the cancer was returning so evidence for theory a. The evidence for theory b 'I am worrying that the cancer has returned was':

- all the professionals whom she spoke to said that was not the case
- she had a lot of trust in her team
- she was under regular review so that they could pick up any problem
- pain was not necessarily a symptom of early cancer return.
- her professionals thought that the pain could be due to nerve damage and needed to be managed in other ways, more likely medication.
- when she was anxious the pain was worse

A complicated issue is that of checking for cancer return, so the principle that should be followed is check the number of times that is evidence based to prevent re-occurrence, and as the health professionals recommend, and attend agreed medical follow-ups. Excessive checking could make the health anxiety worse, and avoidance of checking could miss any re-occurrence.

In terms of evaluating the dangerousness of a particular symptom, as stated earlier, it is helpful to ask, as was mentioned earlier:

- Is this symptom new?
- Is this symptom persistent?
- Is this symptom severe?

If the answer to these questions is yes then it would be wise to attend the GP for assessment, but if the answer is no, then it is reasonable to monitor the symptom. Similarly, if there are a mixture of answers, then more 'yes' answers are more concerning than more 'no' answers. Potentially more frequent checks could slightly increase the chance of picking up an early serious symptom, but there may be a lot of false positives, and the burden of checking will increase anxiety. It is a difficult balance to strike. The other things myself and Jackie worked on was that worrying is a way of avoiding the main issue of accepting that she really had experienced cancer, and that this had various implications for her life: we agreed as a goal to look at these, to help her work on getting full support.

There are similar areas of complexity when patients have other disorders such as neurological and cardiac conditions. A person may be recovering from a myocardial infarction, but start experiencing chest pain which has no medical cause. As always, we would develop a formulation, particularly looking at precipitating factors for the pain. Chest pain is quite a common symptom, probably caused by muscle tension, and can be easily mistaken for cardiac disease pain. The CBT treatment plan would be, as before, addressing and challenging catastrophic thinking, and reducing safety and avoidant behaviours. It may also make sense to try to problem-solve what the stressful events are that are contributing to the symptoms. An additional technique that can be done is discriminating the symptoms of anxiety from those of cardiac disease (or whatever the disease is that the person has), as described here:

| | |
|---|---|
| *Therapist (T):* | one thing we could do would be to help you discriminate between the symptoms of your heart disease and anxiety |
| *Patient (P):* | they seem quite alike |
| *T:* | that might be the case, but there may also be differences. Can you think of why this exercise may be helpful? |
| *P:* | it might reassure me. |
| *T;* | and help you manage anxiety correctly and your heart problem correctly. Perhaps we could draw out two columns on this piece of paper. (Draws these). What are the main symptoms of anxiety? |
| *P;* | I tend to hyperventilate, and I feel a bit sick, occasionally I get chest pain but not always. |
| *T:* | what's it like when you have angina? |
| *P:* | it always happens after exertion like a walk uphill or with cold weather, it's more like a tightness in the chest comes on, I'd struggle to walk. |
| *T:* | would you be able to continue if it was anxiety? |
| *P:* | Yes. |
| *T:* | What tends to happen before anxiety? |
| *P:* | it would be stressful event or a period of worrying. The anxiety would come on much more suddenly. |

We continued to help the patient discriminate the symptoms, he can use this sheet to try to make the best decisions when he has pain (this technique can be used for any medical symptoms).

### Interaction between health anxiety and medically unexplained symptoms

There also exists the situation where the patient has medically unexplained symptoms and health anxiety. In our experience, in most cases of MUS, patients do not catastrophise about their symptoms, the concern is more of the discomfort of the symptoms and the impact on their ability to function. (They may have health anxiety, in the sense that they are preoccupied with symptoms that are not viewed to be medically significant). This view is supported by research, see Rief, Heuser and Fichter (1996). The clinical approach here, if this health anxiety were present, would be to help the patient appraise any symptoms rationally and reasonably.

## General anxiety disorder in LTC

This is a disorder characterised by persistent worry, associated anxiety, and physical symptoms. In a review paper by Culpepper (2009), it is suggested that patients with generalised anxiety disorder approach pain from the perspective of uncertainty, uncontrollability, and unpredictability. Peptic ulcer is 2.8 times greater in patients with generalised anxiety disorder and irritable bowel is more common. Cardiovascular disorders have been associated with this anxiety disorder. Also, 29% of patients with endocrine disorders suffer from GAD and 10–16% of patients with COPD suffer from GAD. From the other direction, it is likely that the development of medical problems will be an activating event for GAD: it is known that patients with this anxiety disorder have an intolerance of uncertainty which can be activated if they face dealing with heart disease, cancer, or other medical problems, with the associated risk to well-being and life itself. So, the GAD formulation is that patients who are dealing with a health problem are likely to worry excessively about it, producing quite a low level chronic anxious arousal which may amplify the symptoms. In the GAD model developed by Robichaud et al. (2019), GAD is believed to be driven by intolerance of uncertainty. Other factors that influence the condition are negative problem orientation, cognitive avoidance, and positive beliefs about worry (e.g. that worry helps you solve problems, or it means you are a good person for worrying).

The approach to treating GAD is to address these maintenance factors. As in this example: Mr Harold was referred to me (PK) for consideration for a course of CBT. Two years prior he had severe depression on the back of two bereavements and ulcerative colitis. He was very ill from the latter and nearly died, and he has been through a rehabilitation process which was going reasonably well. He is left with moderate General Anxiety Disorder. Whenever he gets a symptom, or there is a problem in the family or a stressor, he gets into immediate negative thoughts such as, 'what if I will get ill again', 'what if I won't cope', 'what if I relapse.' He then worries and focuses on his symptoms or problems. Memories become more prominent, and he feels anxious, which intensifies these processes. He then becomes very self-critical, and feels a bit down, worsening the cycle. He tries to micro-manage situations and to be certain about things, and is also somewhat avoidant. In this case I got the patient to work with me on a CBT GAD approach, and we complimented this with a self-help book (Robichaud & Dugas, 2015). He followed the structure in the book: the first section is 'worry awareness', this awareness is increased through keeping a diary, and worries are categorised as actual problems which should be faced, and hypothetical worries which should be acknowledged as such. For example, he sometimes started worrying about whether he would ever get a job, the associated financial implications, the threat to his self-esteem, and the ability to cope with a job. He tended to escalate these worries in a typical GAD manner, with lots of 'what-ifs' such as 'what if this happened . . . what if that happened?' for example, 'what if I can't find a job . . . I'll run out of money . . . I could lose my house . . . my girlfriend will leave if this happens . . . I'll be on the street . . . what if I do get a job . . . what if I can't cope with it' etc. In keeping the diary, it helped him realise that most of these worries were hypotheticals. An actual problem would be something that anyone would recognise as a problem, that it had a potential immediate solution, and it was grounded in real current events. Using this formula, we identified the problem as: 'not having a job but trying to find a way to get one that he could cope with, and paid adequately.' We linked this in to his negative problem orientation, in that he tended to see looking for a job as a problem that was stressful and was avoided: there was a sense that employers may reject him because of his disability, and there may be some truth in this.

He addressed positive beliefs about worry, by listing the reasons why the belief 'I should worry because it helps me solve problems', was not true: the reasons recorded were that you can solve problems without worrying, that worry made you anxious, that it reduced your ability to solve problems, that weighing up the pros and cons of a choice and writing a specific goal was the best way to solve problems. He started to understand the way that intolerance of uncertainty worked: although it was true that he now had some disabilities, such as difficulty walking, and some concentration difficulties, he wanted to be certain that they were not going to impact on his ability to interact with people or do tasks, and this tended to lead to an avoidant position. This was worked on by getting him to embrace uncertainty using behavioural experiments, for example, he agreed to face seeing some friends that he had not seen before, he was unsure how they would react to his current problems, but he associated this uncertainty with a negative outcome. He followed this up with other experiments in facing situations he was unsure of, and reducing seeking verbal reassurance from his girlfriend. The final strategy was addressing cognitive avoidance through exposure. This involved writing a script of his worst fear (of being in a wheelchair, and dependent on others) and this was read repeatedly until habituation to these anxious images occurred.

### What adaptations need to be made to the treatment of GAD when someone has a medical condition?

There does not seem to be specific literature that gives guidance on this; however, our belief is that no significant alterations need to be made to the CBT approaches, and that working to increase intolerance of uncertainty, orienting patients towards solving problems, addressing positive beliefs about worry and imagery exposure are legitimate strategies for the medically ill person with a long-term condition. It may be that interventions from other approaches to GAD such as Borkovec, Robinson, Pruzinsky and DePree (1983) could be used: these would include worry postponement, and this may have some additional utility as some of the worries have more truth in them.

## Panic disorder in long-term conditions

Panic disorder is associated with a range of physical health problems: in asthma the prevalence rate of panic is between 6.5% and 24%, and incidence is high in other respiratory illness (Katon, Richardson, Lozano & McCauley, 2004). Again, there is an association between most types of cardiovascular disease and panic

(Fleet & Beitman, 1998) and an emerging problem is the high rate of panic in patients who have been fitted with an emergency defibrillator. Most studies also show that having panic disorder does lead to smallish increases in cardiovascular disease later in life, though the mechanism is unclear (Fleet & Beitman, 1998). Symptoms of air hunger, breathlessness, suffocation, chest tightness are common in both cardio and respiratory illness and panic disorder, and this may cause errors in diagnosis and treatment.

In the CBT model of panic disorder, the central maintenance factor which gives rise to panic attacks is seen as the catastrophic misinterpretation of bodily sensations. Research evidence shows that individuals with panic disorder more readily detect slight changes in bodily sensations than normal controls, and are more likely to interpret these as threatening (Mathews & Macleod, 1985). Thus, a typical scenario in panic disorder is that the patient may be sitting watching television and suddenly notice their heart fluttering slightly. Most people may not notice such an event in their body (which are quite normal), but for the person predisposed to panic attacks this sensation is perceived as dangerous and evidence that some imminent disaster is about to occur. In this example the patient may have the NAT 'I'm having a heart attack.' Other typical NATS are:

* 'I'm having a stroke'
* 'I'm going to faint/collapse'
* 'I'm going to die'
* 'I'm going crazy'
* 'I'm going to lose control'
* 'I'm going to be sick'
* 'I'm going to wet myself'

If anyone experiences this type of NAT and believes it to a high degree, then they are going to become extremely anxious. This in turn generates further physical symptoms of anxiety (for example breathlessness, palpitations, dizziness; numbness and tingling), that are then taken as further evidence that something catastrophic is about to occur. Certain specific physical symptoms (bodily sensations) tend to generate specific NATS, and making these connections with the patient is important in terms of the CBT interventions that are made. To manage their panic symptoms, the patient may engage in safety seeking behaviours in response to physical symptoms and specific NATS. These can include checking the pulse, controlling breathing, drinking water, going out for fresh air, etc. Some safety behaviours are highly idiosyncratic, and these need to be comprehensively assessed with the patient in order to ensure the optimum treatment outcome. In the patient's mind it is the use of these safety behaviours that prevents the feared catastrophe encapsulated in the NAT, from occurring, and thus are repeated whenever necessary.

The person prone to experiencing panic attacks usually engages in hypervigilant body scanning behaviours. This involves regular mental scanning of the body to monitor for signs of potential panic symptoms, which often in itself is sufficient to trigger a panic attack, hence patients with panic disorder often describing their panic attacks as occurring seemingly 'out of the blue.' Indeed, often one of the most distressing aspects of panic attacks for some patients is the fact they occur in situations such as watching TV or whilst asleep. The triggers to such panic attacks are probably detection of minor changes in internal bodily sensations, which will be more common if you have a medical disorder, that are interpreted as dangerous, thus precipitating an attack. If the patient can work out the typical triggering situations for his panic (e.g. crowds, queues, supermarkets) then he is likely to avoid these situations in the future. This agoraphobia is problematic in that if the person avoids these triggers, he does not learn that his feared catastrophe does not occur, but if he cannot avoid, he is immediately feeling anxious at the thought of facing it and therefore more likely to experience a panic attack.

The standard treatment from a behavioural or cognitive perspective is to help the patient to understand his symptoms, and to recognise that panicky body sensations are not dangerous: one can see that this raises various therapist issues when a patient does have an actual medical disease, such as:

- Understanding the nature of the physical illness that the patient has, helping the patient disentangle physical from panic symptoms
- Considering what, if any, modifications need to be made to the standard CBT approach to panic disorder. Particularly the safety of doing exposure exercises both interoceptive and situational.

So, if a patient has a medical problem and panic disorder, then these factors need to be considered: first of all, the therapist should have assessed whether the person has any medical health problems. Graded exposure programs should be developed in consultation with patients' respiratory physicians or GPs, and only begun after medical treatment has been optimised. The part of therapy that is plainly most challenging is the hyperventilation exercise, so if it was possible to bring about improvements using cognitive restructuring, psychoeducation, and situational exposure, and avoid doing the hyperventilation this may be better and safer. Interoceptive exposure tasks (e.g. planned hyperventilation) can however, be undertaken, but only when patients are not unwell with an infective exacerbation (Livermore, Sharpe & McKenzie, 2010). If patients are having frequent panic attacks anyway, there is a stronger case to do interoceptive exposure because the patient is suffering the effects of the panic attacks anyway

Dialogue to help patient think about treatment planning:

*T:*  When we are thinking about CBT treatment for a panic, we need to know whether you have any physical health problems. Do you?
*P:*  I've got mild COPD, which I think makes the panic worse?
*T:*  How is your COPD now? Do you have any infections?
*P:*  It's relatively mild at the moment, I don't think I currently have any infections

*T:*   The stages of therapy are helping you understand what drives the panic, catastrophic thinking and avoidant behaviour, as we talked about earlier. Later,
we want you to face situations that you are avoiding to help you see whether
they are dangerous or not. We will do this in consultation with your GP. We
could even do it in the GP surgery to be on the safe side. What do you think
of this?

*P:*   I'm not keen on doing the panic provocation, I'm worried I can make my
symptoms worse.

*T:*   I want to collaborate with you in devising the treatment plan. There are things
we can do first and will see how it goes. In the meantime, I'll talk to your GP.

### Panic and asthma

The principal component in the standard CBT treatment of panic attacks is exposure to internal physiological sensations (interoceptive exposure) that are associated with anxiety and panic because of the fear of dyspnoea. Deshmukh, Toelle,
Usherwood, O'Grady and Jenkins (2007) paper, is a thorough review of the
asthma, panic and CBT issues, suggest that interoceptive exposure habituating
patients to dyspnea symptoms may have to be substituted by CBT approaches
such as education, monitoring, and discrimination of symptoms. This is just a
review and it seems that the practical issue as to whether asthma patients should
be given interoceptive exposure has not been researched. Barrera, Grubbs, Huhig
and Teng (2014) review the use of interoceptive exposure with panic and COPD,
and whilst noting that treatments have not used this, they feel that it is a safe technique because exercise is used as part of pulmonary rehabilitation programmes.

Situational exposure exercises seem a bit safer here. If one is using the principles of exposure to typical agoraphobic triggers such as supermarkets, enclosed
places, crowds, etc. on the basis that the anxiety will eventually habituate with
repeated practice.

### Cardiac disease and panic

Similarly, with heart disease, a recent paper has addressed many of these issues
(Tully, Sardinha & Nardi, 2017) with a model called PATCHD: Panic Attack
Treatment in Comorbid Heart Diseases is based on enhancing coping skills, per-
forming safe interoceptive exposures and supervised exercise, and countering
avoidance to reduce panic attack frequency.

### Summary of the use of CBT treatments of panic where there is medical illness

It seems reasonable to use education about models of panic with emphasis on
de-catastrophising, education about disentangling asthma/cardiac symptoms
from anxiety symptoms, and graded exposure exercises to triggers with expected

learning that the anxiety will diminish and is not dangerous. Regarding the use of interoceptive exercises it seems that most studies hold back from incorporating these exercises in to their programmes, but there has been a suggestion that should be included Barrera et al. (2014).

Our suggestion here is that these are reasonable steps to take:

- Initially use standard approach to panic including formulation and the role of catastrophising, discrimination between respiratory disease and anxiety symptoms, coupled with graded exposure exercises to avoided triggers. if this brings about resolution of the panic that is fine.
- If not then consider doing interoceptive exercises in the following way: the therapist is aware of the person's medical condition; the GP has stated that the exercises are safe; the exercises are done in an environment where anything going wrong (however unlikely) could be addressed, for example, in the GP surgery; the exercises start slowly (in contrast to a healthy person where panic can be induced in the first session); the patient is not experiencing an acute exacerbation of cardiac disease, asthma, or COPD; the person is allowed to debrief longer than usual.

It does have to be said that this is a suggestion based on the available literature due to the absence of specific clinical trials.

## PTSD and cancer

It is possible that patients have been so traumatised by their experience of illness that they would meet the criteria for PTSD, indeed the cancer experience qualifies as a particular pathway by which a person may develop PTSD. The prevalence of PTSD symptoms among cancer patients and survivors is around 7.3–13.8% (Cordova, Riba & Spiegel, 2017): there is a large variability in incidence rates of PTSD because of methodological issues, and because of where the person is in their cancer experience. There are a range of potential physical factors that predict vulnerability to PTSD, such as advanced stage, severity of illness, recency of treatment and re-occurrence of illness but the results are not conclusive (Kangas, Henry & Bryant, 2002). The psychological factors that have been identified as making someone vulnerable to PTSD across studies are: prior negative life stressors, a history of psychological disturbance, elevated psychological distress subsequent to the diagnosis, female gender, younger age at diagnosis, lower social economic status and education, emotionally reactive temperament, avoidant coping style, poor social support and social functioning, and reduced physical functioning (Kangas et al., 2002). There are distinctive features of cancer as a stressor including the experience of diagnosis, treatment processes and side effects, its life-threatening nature, etc. The intrusions that patients experience are likely to be more future orientated, arousal symptoms of PTSD may be both effects of the illness or treatment.

### Identification of PTSD and treatment

Screening patients with cancer for PTSD symptoms will alert clinicians to debilitating symptoms such as intrusiveness, physiological arousal and avoidance phenomena, which adversely impact functioning and well-being (Rustad, David & Currier, 2012). Aside from or comorbid with PTSD, it is important for clinicians to be aware that patients may have a range of comorbid anxiety, depressive or substance abuse problems that need to be considered after they have experienced a trauma. (Kangas et al., 2002).

There is evidence that CBT is an effective treatment for cancer related mental health problems, but this is from few studies and this field is under-researched (Dimitrov, Moschopoulou & Korszun, 2019). Kangas, Milross and Bryant (2014) found that CBT was effective in a small group of head and neck cancer patients with PTSD: the core elements used were psychoeducation, Progressive Muscle Relaxation and breathing training, cognitive therapy, in vivo and imaginal exposure (to the worst part of the illness) and activity scheduling. The authors recommend flexibility in the scheduling and application of the programme. The timing of any PTSD treatment would have to be considered in the light of the patient's other treatment schedules and life responsibilities. Consideration needs to be given as to the balance of exposure work, and elements like cognitive restructuring and behavioural change. It may be easier to be treated with an SSRI, but potential drug interactions would suggest that an experienced physician should administer this.

## PTSD and cardiac events

A review has been conducted in to whether it is legitimate to have a diagnosis of PTSD arising from cardiac events: the main findings were that the prevalence of Cardiac Disease Induced-PTSD ranged between 0% and 38% (averaging at 12%) and was highly dependent on the assessment tool used. The most consistent risk factors are of a psychological nature (e.g. pre-morbid distress). Whilst acknowledging concern that there is a sort of 'trauma creep' in which stressors such as health problems are being viewed as traumas, they conclude that their review sheds light on the phenomenon of cardiac disease induced-PTSD, emerging among a small segment of the cardiac-disease patient population. Given the absolute number of cardiac-disease patients around the globe, this 'small segment' effectively adds up to many individuals (both patients and family members), who may be underdiagnosed and undertreated (Vilchinsky, Ginzburg, Fait & Foa, 2017)

## PTSD post-ITU

Some patients have experienced PTSD after intensive care unit (ITU) treatment. Many factors are associated with the development of PTSD in patients, including increased length of stay, and higher levels, and longer duration, of sedation. Patient-related factors associated with a higher risk of PTSD include younger age, being female, previous psychological problems and recall of delusional memories from ICU, in contrast, the formation of even fragmented factual memories may reduce the risk of PTSD. Optimum, analgesia-based sedation may help patients to form factual memories of ICU, so possibly reducing the risk of the PTSD condition arising. Patient diaries, written by health professionals and family members and close friends, may also support patients in coming to terms with traumatic memories, and so reduce their emotional and psychological symptoms (Jones, 2010). At the time of writing, there are many patients who have been in ITU, many with an existing long-term condition, with Covid-19 virus, and it is possible there will be an increase in cases of PTSD after ITU treatment. Psychological treatment, post ITU, may present challenges: patchy memories; hallucinations, ongoing physical problems, avoidance of health triggers, and a distrust of health professionals (Murray et al., 2020). In the case of Covid, a high (50% at the time of writing) death rate, and the occurrence of hypoxia (which may affect memory) will make things extra challenging. However, the Covid patient will be more aware of their admission into ICU, and this may be protective (Murray et al., 2020.)

What are the modifications required to CBT to work with this PTSD ITU group? If the Ehlers and Clark (2000) approach is being used, then the following is recommended:

- psychoeducation and normalising about the ITU experience.
- Individualised case formulation; looking at the role of threatening appraisals of the trauma and its aftermath, the fragmentation of trauma memories, the problematic behavioural and cognitive strategies.
- Reclaiming and rebuilding your life.
- Updating trauma memories through exposure, this can be aided if diaries are kept or family or ICU staff can clarify the narrative. There will need to be focus on 'hotspots' of the most frightening moments, for example the person may think, 'I can't breathe . . . I'm suffocating', and the alternative which can be inserted and integrated into the reliving could be 'It was difficult to breathe because I was on a ventilator, but I can breathe now as the illness has passed, and I can prove this by taking slow deep breaths' (Murray et al., 2020).
- Trigger discrimination can help patients identify the differences between the safe here and now, and the frightening trauma; this is done by writing a list of the differences.
- Revisiting the ITU site in vivo, in imagination, or in Google maps will be part of the treatment.
- Distorted beliefs such as 'These flashbacks mean I'm losing my mind' can be challenged.
- Safety behaviours such as health anxiety type of checking, seeking reassurance and avoidance of medical procedures should be addressed.

## Interaction of phobias and long-term medical conditions

It is possible that patients have phobias that interact with their long-term condition in challenging ways. Patient may have phobias to blood/injury, needles, hospitals, MRI scans, etc., and the avoidance that comes with these phobias may make it difficult for patients to engage with treatment, or may make treatment particularly stressful. Regarding blood injury phobia, the clinical features of this are fainting and sometimes nausea, and fearful avoidance of blood and related objects. It is present in 2–4.5% of children and adults. Sixty-eight per cent of patients have relatives with the same problem, which is three times higher than normal, it therefore shows a high inherited/genetic factor. From an evolutionary perspective, there is likely to be a behaviour of being still/lying flat to preserve blood, (and a freeze response) to deter predators. When the person experiences the triggering situation it is theorised that there is a raise in blood pressure followed by a fall in blood pressure and an associated fainting response. This is called a diphasic response, but it is not accepted that this happens in all blood phobic patients. In a large study Ritz, Meuret and Simon (2013) surprisingly found that only 20% of blood injury patients, compared to 26.6% controls had this response.

The triggering situations are typically: medical procedures, injections, surgery/hospitals, medical programmes, becoming pregnant, the word 'blood', careers in nursing/medicine, descriptions of surgery, etc. Treatment, as with other patients, is exposure, which is graded, prolonged, regular and focused. This is used after the patient is taught 'applied tension' where the patient is asked to tense the muscles in arms, chest and legs for 10–15 seconds (or until a feeling of warmth occurs rising in the face), they then stop tensing for 20–30 seconds and repeat 5 cycles of tension and release five times a day, and this should help them maintain their blood pressure (Ost & Sterner, 1987). This has been shown to be a technique that is easily learned and does protect against fainting (Vögele, Coles, Wardle & Steptoe, 2003). The therapist then provides exposure exercises in the session whilst the patient practices the applied tension, if available, it is a good idea to monitor the patient's blood pressure during these exercises. If the patient feels faint and is likely to faint, it may be better to stop the exercise there, and expose the patient to a lower-level trigger, this because the fainting is aversive and may lead to further avoidance, although it is not dangerous. There can be a problem in accessing blood and related exposure materials, and suggestions are using fake blood (from the joke/theatre suppliers), videos of operations and of blood donations, phlebotomy departments, pricking one's own finger using a sterile needle, imaginary exposure, arranging for the patient to have a blood test, accessing blood in a vial from a hospital or phlebotomist. There are some safety precautions that need to be considered here.

*Needle phobia:* this phobia can interfere with the take up of treatment including vaccination (which may be particularly important with the Covid situation). In a review paper, McLenon and Rogers (2019) showed that most children showed needle fear, while prevalence estimates for needle fear ranged from 20–50% in adolescents and 20–30% in young adults. In general, needle fear decreased with increasing age and both needle fear and needle phobia were more prevalent in females than males. Avoidance of influenza vaccination because of needle fear occurred in 16% of adult patients, 27% of hospital employees, 18% of workers at long-term care facilities, and 8% of healthcare workers at hospitals (this may affect the take up of Covid vaccines). Needle fear was common when undergoing venepuncture, blood donation, and in those with chronic conditions requiring injection. (It is important to ensure when assessing fear of needles that patients are not blood phobic, with a tendency to faint).

Treatment of needle phobia is standard exposure using a behavioural rationale. Again, one has the challenge of obtaining appropriate exposure materials. Possible objects are needles of varying sizes, viewed increasingly closer to the patient, building to the point of holding, touching and describing the needle, holding a needle and syringe on the arm, pricking the patients thumb with a pin prick needle, then imagining a large needle going into the vein and the blood being drawn out, videos of phlebotomy, visiting a phlebotomy or blood donation department. The biggest step for the patient is for them to have blood taken, which can be graded by distraction and looking away at first if necessary. It may be necessary to get this done several times, and it will be essential to get a GP to order this.

### Other anxiety disorders

There is a diagnostic category in DSM-5 called anxiety disorder due to another medical condition. To give this diagnosis to a patient, there must be evidence that shows the anxiety (not better explained by another anxiety disorder or due to delirium), is due to the direct physiologic effects of another medical condition (American Psychiatric Association, 2013) and history, physical examination, or laboratory findings are used to establish this direct effect. Clinically significant distress must be present, and the functioning of the person in social, occupational, or other areas of life must be impaired.

Some of the medical conditions that may be involved in this disorder are hyperthyroidism (high thyroxine), hypothyroidism (low thyroxine), hypoglycemia (low blood sugar) and Cushing's disease (too much cortisone). Heart related problems such as congestive heart failure and arrhythmia may also cause this disorder. Breathing problems such as COPD, pneumonia and hyperventilation also can initiate anxiety. Neurological conditions like encephalitis or neoplasms can lead to anxiety (American Psychiatric Association, 2013).

There are other anxiety disorders including social phobia, OCD but we have not particularly discussed them here, as they do not obviously relate to physical symptoms.

At the time of writing, Covid-19 has resulted in an increase in known risk factors for mental health problems. Together with unpredictability and uncertainty, lockdown and physical distancing might lead to social isolation; loss of income;

loneliness; inactivity; limited access to basic services; increased access to food, alcohol and online gambling; and decreased family and social support, especially in older and vulnerable people (Moreno, Wykes, Galderisi, Nordentoft, Crossley, Jones et al., 2000) Patients may suffer long-term effects of Covid, with the implication for mental health described in Chapter 1. The downturn in the economy caused by the virus will lead to unemployment, financial insecurity and poverty. As resources are directed to Covid other physical problems are not being treated normally. Hospital workers have been exposed to difficult experiences. At the time of writing the longer-term consequences of Covid for anxiety are unknown.

## Chapter summary

There are excellent CBT treatments of health anxiety whether patients do or do not have a long-term condition. The approach will involve challenging thoughts, reducing safety and avoidance behaviours, and building up a credible picture of causes of the symptoms. Generalised anxiety disorder can occur, and can be treated by encouraging tolerance of uncertainty, better problem-solving, challenging positive beliefs about worry and so on. Panic disorder is more common in respiratory and cardiovascular conditions and can be treated using CBT approaches, although careful consideration must be made around interoceptive exposure. PTSD can occur in response to serious medical problems, and stays in ITU, and responds to normal CBT approaches with a focus on reliving. Blood and needle phobias can interfere with medical treatment, but are treatable with exposure approaches.

## Chapter 8

# A different angle

## Helping patients maintaining identities through life story work, social interaction and strengths-based CBT

In this chapter we will consider the impact of having an LTC or MUS on a person's identity. A diagnosis can mark a moment in time when a person experiences a sense of loss of the old and familiar self, transitioning to a new and unknown period of their life that can leave them confused and lost. A dichotomy of the 'before and after' (long-term ill health) can ensue, which can have a severe impact on identity. When seeking to understand issues relating to identity, it is important to explore both the person's individual and social identities. As cognitive behavioural therapists, particularly at a High Intensity level, we are adept at formulating beliefs at the different levels (NATs, rules and core beliefs) about the individual. We work in collaboration to understand the onset and development of the person's belief system that has made them vulnerable to depression and/or anxiety in addition to their LTC or MUS. We may not focus on their roles within different social groups or relationships, but these clearly are important to our identity, more so when feeling isolated, confused and misunderstood following the diagnosis of an LTC or the lack of diagnosis in the case of MUS.

The chapter will begin with a brief overview of the life story approach to identity, which emphasises the importance of the person's stories as a means for understanding who they are (Ryan & Walker, 2016). This is particularly salient in the case of people who have LTC or MUS as it provides an opportunity to place their health condition in the context of their life story, allowing a sense of perspective. This leads to a discussion of how we can focus on the persons' strengths and resilience to maximise the gains from CBT. The importance of social identity and group identification is also examined, as this has been shown to have both psychological benefits and a positive impact on overall well-being in people suffering from chronic health conditions. We will consider the growing evidence which suggests that maintaining connections with social groups, and identification with new groups can reduce symptoms of depression and anxiety associated with LTC (Haslam, Jetten, Cruwys, Dingle & Haslam, 2018). As with other chapters, there will be practical exercises and ideas for interventions and homework tasks, and case examples based on people the authors have worked with. We would hope that this approach can be integrated with a traditional CBT approach.

DOI: 10.4324/9780367824433-11

## Life story approach

Having a sense of who we are is something we can take for granted. But people who use mental health services often find their identity is defined in terms of their diagnosis. This is even more important for someone who has an LTC or MUS, as diagnosis and symptoms become salient frames of reference to their sense of self, and how they perceive others (including healthcare professionals) view them. This can affect their relationships and interactions, within and outside mental health services.

There have been many practical applications of the life story approach within various health and social care contexts, and an examination of these will provide the basis for exploring the ways in which this approach can inform CBT practice in general, and for helping people with LTC to maintain a sense of their identity through changes in health. Life story books were first introduced more than 30 years ago in social service settings for children being placed for fostering and adoption. They were used to ease transitions in care by maintaining a sense of the child's identity (Ryan & Walker, 2007). Now a range of patient groups use them, including older people (Clarke, Hanson & Ross, 2003), people with life-threatening and terminal illnesses (Young & Rodriguez, 2006; Hitcham, 2007), children who have experienced trauma (Rose & Philpot, 2005) and people with learning disabilities (Atkinson, McCarthy & Walmsley, 2000; Hewitt, 2003, 2006b). for a systematic review of the use of life story work in health and social care see McKeown, Clarke and Repper (2006).

A life story book is a biographical account of a person's life. This includes stories of experiences and relationships that have shaped their identity. For example: stories and photographs from childhood, including family relationships, holidays and friends; any significant event in the person's life such as weddings (either own or friends and family), special birthdays and places they have lived (for a detailed account of issues relating to the compilation of life stories see Hewitt (2006a). These are the kinds of things that make us who we are, and is often the kind of information that is looked for in the early experience interview within CBT assessment. In healthcare practice there is often a gap in acknowledging the life history of the person that goes beyond their clinical profile. Information about someone's life experiences and relationships helps us to see an individual in broader terms and emphasises their uniqueness (Hewitt, 2003; Moya, 2009). Recovery and social inclusion philosophy recognise the importance of understanding the individual identities of people who experience mental distress. This is highlighted in the tidal model (Barker, 2001), which focuses on engaging with the person on their own terms, trying to enter their world rather than encouraging them to enter ours. Sometimes this can be difficult, particularly in busy inpatient settings where the information about the person is medically orientated and there are limits on time for meaningful engagement.

### The importance of language

The dominance of the medical model, and the consequences for the perceived identity of the person, have been well documented. Susko (1994) compared two approaches that staff use to people who are labelled mentally ill. These are 'caseness' and 'narrative.' Caseness refers to 'an intellectual construct that facilitates the objectification of a person in the medical system: the person becomes a case' or is primarily perceived as one.' Susko contrasts this to the narrative approach, which 'supports individuals coming to their own voice by allowing their story to unfold and to be told.' Susko suggests that the caseness approach encourages staff to view the person as a patient, whereas the narrative approach looks beyond the patient to viewing the person as an individual with a unique life history. He suggests that the narrative approach empowers the individual by redressing the power disparity inherent in the caseness approach. We ask the reader to reflect whether we always treat people as people rather than cases.

### Life story exercises

There are many ways to use life story methods in therapy. They can be used to encourage engagement, building the therapeutic relationship through developing shared meaning, and a means for increasing person-centred practice by recognising the person as the 'expert' in their own experience. In addition to these general benefits, people with LTC and MUS tend to experience higher levels of chronic pain and fatigue, so there is a need to be creative in how we deliver CBT. Table 8.1 provides some examples of life story exercises at different stages of the CBT process. Most of these are incredibly simple but they can soften the clinical focus and enhance the identity information available.

### Life story methods and potential barriers

We appreciate that these methods may not be familiar to the reader's normal practice. However, they provide a more open and flexible way of applying standard CBT techniques. Change takes time and requires action, and we know that we are drawn to the familiar, so anything new is likely to be avoided. Our advice would be to try them out and experiment with them. Setting a behavioural experiment for yourself to test your predictions would be a good way to introduce something new to your own practice. Monitor how you feel during and after using one of these creative methods, taking account of the reaction by the patient and how this compares to the methods you would normally use in a similar situation.

To facilitate the use of creative methods, it is useful to have some materials available in the session such as the following:

- Coloured paper
- Coloured pens
- Objects and activities that stimulate the senses – essential oils, tactile objects
- Music can be played on phone or other device
- Post it sticky notes
- Flash cards
- Access photos or other images on phone in session

*Table 8.1* Life story exercises

| Stage of therapy | Exercise | Rationale |
| --- | --- | --- |
| Assessment | Favourite colour<br>Ask the person what their favourite colour is. You can share yours with them. | This is a question beyond the clinical information required from the assessment. It is a personal characteristic and it can be used later in therapy. See the following. It also sets you as equal, at that point, rather than being clinician and patient. |
| | Life history show and tell<br>For a homework task between sessions 1 and 2, ask the person to gather some photos and objects that represent their identity. They can present their story in session 2 in their own way. You may need to set some time limit, and navigate the story to keep it focused, but try and go with the flow of the person's story. It is still possible to extract the salient features needed for a formulation. Examples include:<br>Time line<br>Mind map<br>Written narrative<br>Poem<br>Art work<br>Scrap book<br>Favourite colour | The life history interview is an essential part of all CBT assessments, but they can be quite dry. By asking the person to tell their story in their own way they are given more control and allows you to see what they highlight as important experiences. |
| Formulation | When drawing out a formulation or printing them out, use the person's favourite coloured paper. Also, you can have a pot of felt tip pens to use when producing formulation diagrams. | Colour can bring information to life, especially if presented using your favourite colour. It will encourage engagement, by reducing the 'black and white' presentation of the diagram as colour is more stimulating visually. |

*(Continued)*

*Table 8.1* (Continued)

| Stage of therapy | Exercise | Rationale |
|---|---|---|
| | Illness stories<br>Use creative methods to explore early experiences of illness. This can include:<br>Photos<br>Art work<br>Piece of music<br>Empty chair exercise (playing self and parent or healthcare professional) | Early experiences of illness are clearly important for the formulation. Making the methods fluid, and giving more control to the person in terms of how they tell their stories will make this less threatening. |
| Treatment & relapse prevention | Creative methods<br>For every intervention you can use a range of creative methods to suit the individual's needs. For example:<br>Develop a metaphor for the impact of the LTC (or MUS) that makes sense to the person, and encourage them to use this to describe and update their journey towards recovery (e.g. the hare and the tortoise story to recognise how the 'all or nothing' rule can be adapted to 'little and often')<br>Role plays and empty chair exercises to challenge the 'sick role' or illness behaviours contributing to the distress<br>Use of 'post-it' stickers on the formulation to emphasise flexibility of movement (e.g. my NATs about my illness in one situation do not necessarily generalise to all situations)<br>Flashcards to capture learning points at every stage of therapy | People with LTC and MUS are more likely to experience fatigue and chronic pain, which makes engagement more challenging to maintain. Making methods varied and creative can reduce the information 'load' required to focus attention. Creative methods can also give a sense of being more in control as you are given choice over how you complete therapy tasks. |

For a useful and accessible guide to using life story methods, see Ryan and Walker (2016), and the series of creative workbooks for CBT produced by Jennifer Guest (2015, 2020).

All the examples presented in the table have one thing in common, the person remained in control of the process of telling their stories. This is vital in order to strengthen the therapeutic bond and to ensure that the person feels not only listening to, but heard.

Table 8.2 Examples of how life story methods were used with people presenting with long-term conditions or medically unexplained symptoms, with co-morbid mental health problems.

| Person | Presenting problem | How life story methods were used in therapy | Comments |
|---|---|---|---|
| HK | Recovering from breast cancer, following a double mastectomy and breast reconstruction. She had difficulty relating to herself, and saw her identity as problematic. She would say 'I am not me anymore.' This caused symptoms of both anxiety (she had a history of GAD), and depression – mourning the loss of her perceived 'old self' prior to cancer and the surgery. | We used photographs in a therapeutic way, to help her to update her image and beliefs about herself. I (HM) asked her to collect a sample of photos over time, including ones she liked and ones she was more critical of. Laying them out in chronological order helped her to see that when she thinks back to a time before the cancer, she is only remembering the times when she believes she looked good and was happy. By having other photos, she did not like of herself, at the same period of time, she could recognise that it is not as black and white. Likewise, there were photos that have been taken since the surgery that she quite liked of herself. For example, she had lost weight and her hair had grown back softer since chemotherapy. We also used the photos in a survey, asking people to describe all the photos using three key descriptors, and there was no difference in the descriptions in terms of positive or negative comments. She was viewed as equally attractive before and after the cancer episode. | Following these interventions, HK had a noticeable shift in her view of herself. The self-critical thoughts reduced and she adopted a more positive and self-compassionate dialogue with herself. This translated into other positive changes, such as getting her hair done and buying new clothes. |
| JS | He had incurred a brain injury many years ago and had chronic depression and symptoms of PTSD. He found it extremely difficult to feel or discuss his emotions. When experiencing a strong sensation like heart racing or a tension headache, | Initially in therapy it took several sessions to build up his confidence enough to engage in the CBT interventions. I used life story approach to model the diverse ways he could tell his story and connect with his past. I used metaphors, including one about a vase, to tell a recovery story. It describes how someone who went through a crisis | JS could tell his story at his own pace, layering it up, and helping him when he didn't have the words, by using metaphors. |

(Continued)

Table 8.2 (Continued)

| Person | Presenting problem | How life story methods were used in therapy | Comments |
|---|---|---|---|
| | he would try and block any associated emotion from escalating by mental avoidance. He would try to suppress his thoughts and distract himself until the feelings passed. This cycle was continuous for many years. | felt broken, but piece by piece began to rebuild themselves, and developed into a mosaic which was stronger than the original vase. This really resonated with him and he slowly began to tell his story and engage fully in CBT. | |
| CN | Presented with GAD and symptoms of Fibromyalgia. She described herself as a perfectionist, and had the 'all or nothing' thinking and behaviour styles associated with perfectionism. She had been very successful in her teaching career but had been out of work for several months due to her health issues. She was a highly intelligent and creative woman. | Between the initial assessment and the follow-up session, I explained to her that we would be exploring her earlier life experiences and she could tell her story how she wanted to. We went through some options and she stated that she liked doing mind maps, so she prepared one for the session as homework. The mind map was very informative and the most interesting feature was how she told her story, and where she placed the most emphasis. The first strand of the mind map she referred to was schooling and education, which shows the importance of this aspect of her life history. | By telling her story in her own way, CN remained in control of the process. She used a mind map to help her to tell her story in a meaningful way, which may not have occurred in a traditional CBT life story interview. |

A life story approach helps the person to contextualise their LTC, giving control over the narrative they produce in relation to their overall identity. This allows for a re-focusing of attention to some of the strengths and positive characteristics which may have become overshadowed since their diagnosis. The next section expands on this by considering a turn to a more strengths-based focus for CBT treatment informed by a positive psychology paradigm.

## Strengths-based CBT models

There has been a movement towards addressing positive aspects of a person's psychology, as opposed to focusing solely on perceived deficits or negative beliefs and behaviours. Beckian Cognitive Therapy has been criticised for this emphasis on 'dysfunctional' beliefs and 'unhelpful' behaviours, with a clear psychopathology that understands the emotional 'problem' as something that manifests in these patterns of thoughts and behaviours. Later iterations of Cognitive Therapy, namely that proposed by Kuyken (2008) and Padesky and Mooney (2012) has attempted to redress this deficit by including positive information in the formulation from assessment, in order to build resilience from the positive resources already available to the individual. It is interesting to note the radical departure made by Seligman in his earlier work (Seligman & Beagley, 1975) on learned helplessness to his later work on positive psychology (Seligman & Csikszentmihalyi, 2014) with a recognition of strength and motivation to change even in the most adverse of circumstances. This is very fitting when applied to people who have been living with LTC and MUS. Over time they can become demoralised and hopeless, and indeed feel they have no control over their bodies and symptoms, despite fighting and trying many different strategies.

Padesky and Mooney (2012) introduced the Personal Model of Resilience (PMR) as a four-stage model to help clinicians work with patient strengths during CBT treatment. The four stages are:

1 Activate past experiences of resilience.
2 Delineate a personal model of resilience strategies that were useful to overcome past obstacles.
3 Apply those strategies to a problem area.
4 Generalise them to different areas of life.

More recently, this model has been tested in a clinical trial comparing its delivery in face-to-face versus internet modality. Victor, Krug, Vehoff, Lyons and Willutzki (2018) found that in a population of college students suffering moderate psychosocial stress, the PMR provided positive outcomes for both face-to-face and internet versions, with face to face being slightly more effective.

A strengths-based approach to CBT would lend itself to LTC (possibly MUS), because by building on the person's strengths and resilience the focus is much more likely to instil hope and encourage engagement. This makes the person the 'expert' on their condition and how they can overcome some of the obstacles they are currently facing. There are several stages to developing a strengths-based approach. Ways to identified strengths are to focus on positive, non-problem based, activities that the person does regularly: we then ask about challenges that they have doing these activities, and what strengths they use to overcome those challenges. Examples of strengths could be commitment, resilience, sense of humour, persistence, ability to seek help etc. and it is important to discover as many strengths as possible. The next stage is to build a 'personal model of resilience-PMR' (Padesky & Mooney, 2012): example of this is to try to turn specific positive things that the person did into more general principles, using metaphors if possible. So the therapist comments 'you've been telling me that you regularly visit your daughter even otherwise you don't always feel like it, and you've got pain. That's amazing. What quality do you think this represents? Are you quite determined? Do you show resilience? Are you loyal? Are you focused on your family? Which of the strengths can you use at the moment, can we write this down and add to your personal model of resilience?' Once the PMR is constructed, the patient is asked to consider how it could help maintain resilience in areas of difficulty. Common challenges in problem areas are considered and written down. The therapist asks the person to scan their PMR for ideas of what might help them persist in the face of obstacles and/or accept aspects of the situation that cannot be changed, the focus is on staying resilient in the face of difficulties rather than success in solving or overcoming them. (Padesky & Mooney, 2012). The final stage is practice, where the person conducts a behavioural experiment to test out your ability to show your strength in that area. The debriefing process focuses on how much they're able to do that and how they can do it more in the future.

## Social identity and the importance of others

So far, we have only considered issues relating to the individual with regard to identity. This fits nicely with a CBT model as it resonates with the formulation developed in therapy. We are now going to consider the individual's identity in relation to others. This requires an examination of theory informed by psychology, in particular the social identity approach and its relevance to the experience of health and mental health problems (Haslam et al., 2018). We begin with a brief overview of the traditional psychological approaches used to understand long-term conditions, which are often described as Chronic Physical Health Conditions (CPHC) within the psychological literature.

The social identity approach moves beyond an understanding of individual differences between people, to understanding how interaction and identification with others can impact on the experience of LTC. We have already established that stress management and acceptance are key issues that need to be addressed when working with people with LTC and MUS, so we now consider these within the social identity model. We have stated the particular importance of the therapeutic relationship when working with people with LTC and MUS. In their study of people with cerebral palsy, Read, Morton and Ryan (2015) found that healthcare professionals often stigmatise patients by use of stereotyping. This can lead to the patient 'enacting' their illness identity in order to fit their healthcare professional's expectation. The similarity or difference of social identities between healthcare provider and patient can also influence care. This was shown by St Claire and Clucas (2012), who found that doctors tended to use an 'us' and 'them' identity classification according to how similar they perceived the class of the patient to their own. This echoes the earlier work of Pendleton and Boschner (1980) in their classic study which showed that doctors spent more time in consultation with patients they perceived as being from an upper-middle class background, as opposed to those with a perceived lower socio-economic status. To help reduce this bias or effect it is important, as health care professionals, that we can look beyond the 'patient' identity and view them more widely in terms of other identities they own. Mathers, Jones and Hannay (1995) found that people who are frequent users of healthcare services are perceived by doctors as being the most demanding and difficult type of patient, which impacts on patient satisfaction. This links back to the work, cited earlier, by Susko (1994) on the caseness and narrative approaches to care relationships. Even knowing a bit of information about the patient beyond their physical and mental health condition helps the healthcare professional to identify with them as a person and not just their diagnosis.

Cruwys, Wakefield, Sani, Dingle and Jetten (2018) examined a sample of 'frequent attenders' of healthcare services. They found that social isolation was a greatest predictor of frequent attendance than any other factor, including severity of symptoms. They implemented an intervention to increase social group membership and noted a significant reduction in frequency in GP attendance over a three-month period. The key observation here is that group membership had to be 'meaningful' to the person. It was not just any group that caused these positive effects. Social connectedness has also been shown to be a good predictor of longevity (Holt-Lundstad, Robles & Sbarra, 2017). More specifically, group identification predicts better outcomes with people with LTC in terms of symptom management and perceived quality of life. This has been demonstrated in different patient populations including heart disease (Haslam, O'Brien, Jetten, Vormedal & Penna, 2005). multiple sclerosis (Wakefield, Bickley & Sani, 2013), and cancer (Harwood & Sparks, 2003). In a meta-analysis of interventions to reduce loneliness across the age spectrum, Masi, Chen, Hawkley and Cacioppo (2011) found that group-based interventions were significantly more effective than one-to-one. As previously stated, not just any group, it must be a group that fosters social identification. Group interventions are more effective when they attend to social processes in addition to cognitions and behaviours. Meaningfulness of the group identification cannot be assumed so, for example, assuming that a group for older people will be effective just based on age of the person. When groups lose their meaning, purpose and function, the protective factor declines. Haslam et al. (2018) hypothesise that the more social identities a person has access to, the more psychological resources they can draw upon, leading to increased benefits to their overall physical and mental health.

## Groups 4 Health programme

In response to the evidence presented so far, Haslam et al. (2018) describe the development of their programme that encourages identity-based connectedness to others. This is called Groups 4 Health. They describe it as a social cure for many problems that result in physical or mental distress. The Groups 4 Health programme encourages both the strengthening or reconnecting with valued existing social identities, and scaffolding the development of new social identities.

The Groups 4 Health programme comprises five modules, which are called the 5 S's (see Table 8.3), and it is a manualised course providing the facilitator with the rationale, evidence base and detailed instructions for how to deliver it. There is a facilitator manual (Haslam et al., 2016a), and a workbook for participants (Haslam et al., 2016b).

This course encourages the use of creative methods, such as network mapping with post-it notes to help the person to recognise existing connections, and where new ones could be targeted. The group itself is used as a resource for modelling the benefits of connecting in groups. It incorporates a relapse prevention element and follow-up session to check maintenance of therapeutic gains. Haslam et al. (2016c) provide impressive evidence of positive evaluation of the programme in terms of tangible improvements, an identifiable mechanism of change, and feasibility to both facilitators and participants. The mechanism of change from this programme is suggested to be social identification. Bearing these benefits in mind, how can we apply this evidence to working with people with LTC and MUS? Well clearly, we need to take account of their existing group affiliations, their values and the opportunities to join new networks. It is important to be mindful of not making assumptions of which groups may appeal. For example, groups based on the physical or mental difficulties they are experiencing may or may not be attractive to the person based on how stigmatising these associations may be to the individual. For some people, a self-help network will provide validation and support from people experiencing similar difficulties. It will depend on how strong the social identification is to that aspect of their identity.

Table 8.3 Groups 4 health

| | |
|---|---|
| 1. Schooling | Raising awareness of the value of groups for health and how to harness them |
| 2. Scoping | Developing social maps to identify existing connections and areas for social growth |
| 3. Sourcing | Training skills to maintain and utilise existing group networks and reconnect to values groups |
| 4. Scaffolding | Using the group as a platform for new social connections and to train effective engagement |
| 5. Sustaining | Reinforcing key messages and troubleshooting (held one month later as a booster session) |

## Chapter summary

This chapter has considered issues relating to identity and how an understanding of these can help the therapeutic relationship and process. We have considered identity from the individual perspective and presented some creative ideas, based on the life story approach, to help the person tell their story in their own way. The strengths-based model builds on this, by highlighting existing strengths and resilience we can use in therapy. We have also presented theory on social identification, and how group identification can help reduce distress associated with both physical and psychological symptoms.

# Part III

# A formulation approach to medically unexplained symptoms

## Chapter 9

# Making sense of MUS, through a formulation approach

## Chapter contents

In this chapter we will briefly outline some of the challenging issues, before presenting practical ideas as to how to adapt CBT to help patients with MUS. The chapter will cover the following: definition, impact and terminology related to MUS, overview of the common conditions or symptoms that typically fall under this umbrella term, treatment approaches to managing these symptoms, and in what setting they are seen. In following chapters there will be a more detailed discussion of how CBT can be used and adapted when treating people with MUS, using some creative ideas, and presenting real case examples from our own practice in a UK Secondary care Specialist service, where the authors have worked.

## Definition, impact and terminology

As described in chapter one MUS refer to a focus on physical bodily sensations, such as pain or fatigue, that cause intense psychological distress and problems functioning. It is believed that patients with MUS form 20% new primary care consultations (Jadhakhan, Lindner, Blakemore & Guthrie, 2019) and Chew-Graham et al. (2017) estimates that the cost to the NHS is almost £3 billion, which makes up almost 10% of the total NHS expenditure. Moreover, the distress and stress caused by MUS to the person can lead to limited quality of life, reduced opportunities for occupation and recreational activities, and can put pressure on relationships. In addition to these personal daily challenges, people who have MUS often form negative beliefs about the medical profession and doctors when they are told that there is nothing 'physically' wrong with them (Wileman, May & Chew-Graham, 2002).

We have chosen to use the term *Medically Unexplained Symptoms (MUS)* throughout this book, as this is the term which has the most longevity in the UK healthcare services. However, there are other expressions currently used in the UK and internationally, such as functional syndromes and psychosomatic disorders, somatisation and Bodily Distress Disorder (Fink & Schröder, 2010) so it is useful to present these variations in order to clarify whether they all refer to

DOI: 10.4324/9780367824433-13

the same concept. Marks and Hunter (2015) conducted a survey amongst people with a medically unexplained presenting problem and found the preferred term by patients was Persistent Physical Symptoms (PPS), but this does not seem to have become commonplace. In this chapter we are taking the position that MUS encompasses patients described as body distressed, functional, psychosomatic, functional syndromes, etc.

## Challenges in understanding MUS

MUS have disconcerted the medical profession, mental health professionals and patients alike for many years. Because they do not neatly fall into a particular category, pathology or psychopathology, patients and healthcare professionals are left in a state of uncertainty as to how to manage or treat these symptoms. Kirmayer and Taillefer (1997) highlight the origins of our understanding of these conditions as part of the ancient philosophical concept of Mind-Body Dualism, where processes and issues relating to the mind and body have been split and understood as parallel processes and systems, and it could be argued that modern medicine continues this approach with specialities divided by bodily systems (cardiology, nephrology, etc.). This dualism contrasts with conceptualisations, within areas of Health and Social psychology, Behavioural Medicine and CBT, where interconnections and integration of the systems are acknowledged. Over the past 30 years there has been attempts to understand this phenomenon, with research and clinical trials conducted worldwide, however interpreting this research is not easy due to a number of issues, including different terminology, conceptualisations and theoretical persuasion. Developing understanding has led to MUS now being considered to be affected by psychological processes and emotional distress. This is difficult to prove in terms of a clear mechanism of symptom generation, as we can only infer this from patient history, illness behaviour and social circumstances (Kirmayer, 1999).

## Some relevant research

One area of healthcare where MUS have been studied widely is Neurology. This is due to the high volume of referrals from GPs based on the nature and presentation of some of the common functional/MUS symptoms, including pain, sensory disturbances and seizure-like activity. Reuber Pukrop, Bauer, Derfuss and Elger (2004) suggest that neurologists are not always sympathetic or responsive to the emotional needs of the patients presenting with MUS. How their clinical views are communicated is crucial for the engagement and outcomes of the patient, and they suggest that there is a need for collaboration and a multi-disciplinary approach between neurologists, (liaison) psychiatrists, psychologists and psychological therapists, and GPs. Kirmayer, Groleau, Looper and Dao (2004) highlight the importance of the doctor-patient relationship, and found that even in the absence of a medical explanation, an acknowledgement of the patient's suffering can reduce stress and increase acceptance of uncertainty (in a Canadian health-care setting): they emphasise the importance of allowing the person to construct their own narrative to make sense of their symptoms, and how social context is an important factor in this. Only when the patient accepts that there is no medical explanation for their symptoms can they be prepared to consider psychological treatments. So, from this research we can see that building a good alliance with patients and colleagues is important.

Due to the wide variance in illness behaviours and presenting symptomology, it has been difficult to develop a unified approach to understanding these disorders. Henningsen, Zipfel and Herzog (2007) suggested a stepped care model for the management of FSS in Germany, ranging from uncomplicated to complicated presentations, with doctor involvement increasing with increasing complexity of presenting symptoms. This model offers a combination of physical and psychological interventions that range from advice on graded activation or exercise, through to individual psychotherapy and a combination of multi-disciplinary interventions. Again, the doctor-patient relationship is identified as essential in the prediction of positive outcomes. This approach is akin to what is typically done in IAPT, so this research suggests that stepped care is important.

Creed et al. (2013) conducted a population-based study of 990 UK adults with a FSS including chronic widespread pain (CWP), irritable bowel syndrome (IBS) or chronic fatigue (CF). Of these, over 50% experienced multiple somatic symptoms. They found that multiple somatic symptoms were associated with more impaired health status both at baseline and at follow-up. Chew-Graham et al. (2017) emphasises the impact MUS has on the healthcare system. GPs can feel a sense of powerlessness, which can impact on the doctor-patient relationship. This is echoed in secondary care in a study of junior doctors who reported either over investigating or avoidance, due to the challenging nature of MUS (Yon, Habermann, Rosenthal, Walters, Nettleton, Warner & Buszewicz, 2017). As already stated, the therapeutic relationship is important for engagement and good outcomes, so being believed and offered support with a clear rationale is essential for patients. Again, Chew-Graham et al. (2017) concludes that a multidisciplinary approach is necessary for effective management of patients with MUS, including professionals from medical and psychology professions in order to provide an integrated service. She highlighted the need to be open-minded and creative in clinical interventions. A recent study has considered which interventions are most helpful with medically unexplained symptoms, and 15 change mechanisms were identified. Those receiving the most consistent support included increasing symptom acceptance, development of coping strategies and positive treatment expectations, although the last mechanism was investigated in only two studies. Almost all mechanisms received support for at least one type of outcome, either at post-treatment or at follow-up (Pourová, Klocek, Řiháček & Čevelíček, 2020).

Again, this is research that backs up multidisciplinary working and stepped care and indicates potential strategies.

## Common MUS presentations and processes

There are many conditions and symptoms that fall under the umbrella term of MUS and there is a table in Chapter 1 summarising this. The most common presentations one is likely to see are: Chronic Fatigue Syndrome (CFS); Fibromyalgia (FM); Irritable Bowel Syndrome (IBS); Non-epileptic seizure disorder (NEAD); and Chronic pain or paralysis without a physical explanation. As stated in the preceding discussion, there is a debate regarding whether it is more effective to treat presenting problems as specific 'conditions' like those listed (e.g. FM), or to treat them using a more transdiagnostic approach. Chalder and Willis (2017) reviewed various treatment conceptualisations and described them as 'splitting' (focusing on the disorder specific presentations) and 'lumping', which espouses treating the main somatic symptoms across the presentations, and they conclude by supporting a transdiagnostic approach, as it is theoretically informed and efficient. The overlapping of common symptoms has been highlighted by Petersen (2020) who found overlapping of FSS/MUS to a prevalence of 9.3% in a Danish population, with little single 'pure' type presentation. This supports work by Deary et al. (2007) and Spence and Moss-Morris (2007) who identified common processes that increase symptoms and disability. These include avoidance of activity, attentional focus on bodily sensations, and an 'all or nothing' thinking style. Fatigue, pain and sleep problems are also common in many MUS presentations.

## Woolford and Allen research

Woolfolk and Allen (2007) developed their Affective Cognitive behavioural Therapy (ACBT) model for somatisation as a 10-session manualised individual CBT approach. The model was informed by evidence from CBT protocols for several other anxiety disorders and depression but it also acknowledges the tendency of people with somatic symptoms to have difficulty recognising and expressing emotions, alexithymia (see Chapter 10), and the social identity process leading to the assignment of the 'sick role' (see Chapter 11). Their original protocol incorporated the following key elements:

- Relaxation techniques to reduce stress
- Behavioural Activation (BA) and communication skills to minimise the 'sick role'
- Training in emotional awareness
- Cognitive restructuring to modify dysfunctional cognitions

They trialled this protocol and showed its effectiveness, but they found that a more individualised approach, with an emphasis on emotional awareness, acceptance and expression, was more effective in the longer term than rigid adherence to the protocol.

The authors believe that people with MUS tend to relapse quickly due to the rigidity of their rules for living, which will pull them back to an 'all or nothing' pattern of thinking and behaviours and this also makes protocol driven interventions challenging. *A CBT formulation driven approach is therefore recommended,* as it acknowledges some common features but addresses the individual nuances of the person's lived experience of having a MUS condition.

## Deary et al. approach

Deary et al. (2007) performed a narrative literature review of the available evidence for a CBT approach to treating MUS. They state that one of the key features of the CBT model is the recognition of symptoms as being autopoietic – that they are autonomous and self-maintaining in a vicious cycle of cognitions, behaviours and physiological elements and that this provides a hypothesis for a novel mechanism for the generation of physical symptoms in the absence of physical pathology or psychopathology (Deary et al., 2007).

*Predisposing factors:* the evidence for genetic predisposition to MUS is poor, but association with particular personality traits has been recognised. In their review, Deary et al. (2007) found a high association of trait neuroticism (meaning a lifelong tendency to experience negative affect), across studies. Perfectionism is also widely associated with MUS, with the characteristic 'all or nothing' thinking and behaviours, (Chalder & Willis, 2017 suggest that this can initially be used positively to help engagement in CBT and support recovery). Early experience of illness behaviour in childhood by self or parents is another key predisposing factor (Craig, Drake, Mills & Boardman, 1994). Hotopf (2003, 2004) suggests that interpersonal behaviour between doctors and patients with MUS is comparable to that of a parent with a sick child so as cognitive behavioural therapists we need to be self-aware of our interactional style to avoid collusion with this parental role in therapy.

*Precipitating factors:* in their review, Deary et al. (2007) found unanimous support of the hypothesis that life events precipitate MUS. This can be explained, in part, due to the prolonged activation of the physiological stress response to life events.

*Perpetuating factors:* Deary et al. (2007) recommend understanding the interactive factors, so the authors would suggest that a judgement is made after assessment as to which of the pertinent factors are most important in driving the symptoms, and a collaborative plan is made with the patient to address these as summarised in this table, and discussed in the separate chapters.

## Treatment setting

Traditionally, in the UK, people presenting with MUS would be treated in specialist services within Secondary Care settings. This would entail long waiting times and the need for augmented physical interventions such as medication whilst

*Table 9.1* MUS factors

| Maintenance factor | Possible strategy |
| --- | --- |
| • *Sensitisation* where there is a heightened physiological and behavioural response to aversive stimuli that has been previously met. | Helping the person to not avoid because of this process, to take constructive steps to lean in to the symptom and to experience it in better ways (Chapter 10) |
| • The HPA axis (hypothalamus pituitary adrenal) is part of the body's response to *stress*. | Help the person reduce the stress in their lives (Chapter 10) |
| • *Attentional processes* | Help the person shift their attention in a helpful way (Chapter 11) |
| • *Attribution* | Help the person address thoughts, rules and beliefs (Chapter 11) |
| • *Behavioural responses:* | Help the person address unhelpful behaviour (Chapter 10) |
| • *Sleep* | Aid them to sleep better (Chapter 11) |
| • *Emotional factors* | Help with emotional awareness, expression, regulation and tolerance (Chapter 12) |
| • *Medication* | Assist patients to use medication rationally (Chapter 9) |
| • *Substance abuse* | Encourage them to not use harmful substances (Chapter 9) |
| • *Secondary gain/fear of recovery* | End secondary gain/fear of recovery (Chapter 13) |

awaiting psychological therapy. On entering these services, it is likely that treatment would be spread over an extended period of time due to the complexity and chronic nature of the problems. The current context, within the UK, has changed with the developments within the IAPT programme (see Chapter 1). People with a range of MUS, are now able to access primary care services for psychological therapy input. We are going to compare and contrast some of the issues related to treatment plans within these two types of service.

It may be assumed that a 'specialist' service would be the best place to treat problems associated with MUS. However, this is problematic for many reasons. We have already established that there is no one universally agreed definition or conceptualisation of MUS, which makes placement in a service challenging. GPs are normally the first healthcare professionals that people approach, so their knowledge and attitudes towards MUS will be pivotal in terms of whether a referral is made to secondary care, and to which service the referral is made. Options include; pain clinics, neurology, psychology, psychological medicine or services for specific presentations such as fibromyalgia or CFS. Once referred, there is often a long wait to be seen and assessed due to the mismatch between supply and demand. Depending on the service, treatment options are likely to be varied. Unlike other presenting problems, such as depression and anxiety disorders, that have NICE guidelines for CBT treatment, there are no such clear guidelines for treating MUS. A CBT formulation driven approach with this patient group requires highly skilled practitioners who are likely to deliver CBT over a longer period of time than other presenting problems. Core skills and meta-competencies are essential for effective CBT treatment. Key areas include:

* Therapeutic relationship
* Collaboration
* Clear and realistic goals
* Conceptual integration of the CBT model
* Psycho-education
* Managing avoidance
* Pacing
* Monitoring outcomes through feedback and regular reviews
* Good relapse prevention
* Managing the ending of therapy

Pacing of therapy may be slowed down in secondary services, as a number of sessions may be more flexible in comparison to Primary Care or IAPT services: whilst this allows time to target more complex issues, it runs the risk of therapist drift. More recently, since the introduction of IAPT services in the UK in 2008, CBT is being delivered in primary care settings. Although initially aimed at treating depression and anxiety disorders, these services have broadened their remit to include LTC and other presenting problems that are characterised by psychological distress, but clearly the treatment length in primary care is limited. Originally, the course of therapy would be informed by the NICE guidelines in terms of recommended treatment length within the disorder specific protocols. However, over time the business models applied within IAPT services has blurred these boundaries and currently there are many services that cap treatment at 6–8 sessions. As we have established, assessment alone for someone presenting with MUS can take two sessions to produce an adequate formulation, and even more to thoroughly engage the person and socialise them to the CBT model, so this clearly leaves little scope for treatment.

Despite the time limitations within IAPT services, we suggest that one approach is that MUS can be treated effectively if broken down into specific problems which can be targeted in separate courses of treatment. By prioritising the problems and focusing on one at a time, symptom relief is possible in a brief period (Rimes, Papadopoulos, Cleare & Chalder, 2014). For example, if someone is presenting with fibromyalgia and have symptoms of depression, you still need a thorough assessment and formulation, but the depression can be treated using BA to help with functioning and pacing of activities. Once the person realises some

*Table 9.2* IAPT and secondary care approaches to MUS

| Secondary care | IAPT |
| --- | --- |
| Longer term treatment based on therapist clinical judgement is normally offered | Limited treatment time, dictated by service model |
| Therapeutic relationship is central to therapy gains, and more time is available for this | Techniques and engagement are central to therapy gains |
| Waiting time for assessment can be many months | Waiting time for assessment can be weeks |
| Long-term CBT can allow for more thorough treatment, but may lead to therapist drift | Short-term model stays focused on symptom relief |
| Motivation may wane over a lengthy period of time | Multiple short-term courses of CBT can help to maintain focus and motivation |
| One therapist throughout | Possibly multiple therapists, which may be an advantage or disadvantage depending on therapeutic bond |

gains from a short course of CBT, they may be more likely to return for further treatment to target other aspects of their problem. This may be to address perfectionism in the form of 'all or nothing' rules or self-critical thinking with a more compassion-focused approach. With each separate treatment course layers of the problems can be addressed, and earlier gains will be reinforced.

Clearly, the message in the book is that no one size fits all when it comes to LTC and MUS. Table 9.2 compares the longer-term treatment offered in secondary care with the short-term model offered in primary care IAPT services.

Sometimes with MUS it is difficult to arrive at a formulation, or it may take some time to evolve: in this case we need to be guided by the goals that have been collaborated on by patient and therapist. The following chapters will look at some techniques to use once an understanding of the problem has been obtained.

## Chapter summary

MUS are common, and challenging for all concerned. Common presentations are chronic fatigue syndrome, fibromyalgia, IBS, non-epileptic seizures and chronic pain or paralysis. There is some debate as to whether to approach these individually, but we believe a transdiagnostic formulation-based approach is best. Maintenance factors will include sensitisation, stress, attention, attribution, behavioural processes, sleep, emotional factors, education and substance use and fear of recovery. These need to be assessed and targeted, either in primary care, perhaps in a staged approach, or in a secondary care setting.

## Chapter 10

# CBT from the inside out

## A lived experience account

This chapter provides a personal account of how one of the authors, Helen Moya, has used CBT to understand and manage symptoms related to Chronic Fatigue Syndrome (CFS) and Irritable Bowel Syndrome (IBS). A brief history of these problems, when and how they manifest, their impact, and how they relate to her overall formulation will be presented. The account is an example of how self-reflection and the use of CBT from the inside-out (Bennett-Levy, Thwaites, Haarhoff, & Perry, 2015) can be used to deepen our understanding of the lived experience of our patients and inform CBT practice.

The self-reflection in this chapter begins with a narrative account of the two conditions I was diagnosed with and how they impacted on my life. A brief formulation of my beliefs, particularly the rules for living, will be used to understand how I responded to stress in unhelpful ways that actually maintained the emotional distress associated with these conditions. Through applying CBT from the inside-out, I develop a more behavioural approach using a functional analysis to respond differently to stress in my daily life. In a timely examination of a recent relapse, during the Covid-19 pandemic, I describe how this approach has freed me from falling into old responses to stress and the associated activation of unhelpful negative beliefs and emotional responses. I finish with an account of how mindfulness practices and self-compassion have kept me in remission and serve as relapse prevention measures.

## Background history

### IBS

I was diagnosed with IBS in 1992 at the age of 25. I had trained as a Registered Nurse for people with Learning Disabilities (RNLD) and was studying for a Psychology degree. I had always been diligent and hard-working, and funded myself through my degree whilst still working as a Staff Nurse in a community hospital.

Initial presentation included constant abdominal bloating, cramping pains and gastric disturbances. I managed these symptoms initially, but over months the condition became chronic and I sought medical advice. I was asked to keep

DOI: 10.4324/9780367824433-14

a diary of dietary intake, daily weighing and girth measurements morning and evening. Interestingly, this data showed significant changes in weight and waist measurement across a 24-hour period that could not be explained by diet. IBS was diagnosed and initial treatment was medication – Colpermin (concentrated peppermint oil, now available over the counter) and mebeverine hydrochloride (antispasmodic for stomach cramps), neither of which provided any noticeable long-term symptom relief.

There would be times when I felt better, and these appeared to be random, but on closer inspection were associated with periods of reduced situational stress – such as during holidays from work and study. During times of increased stress, my attention would be solely focused on my stomach, noticing every little gurgle or sensation. I would constantly check my stomach by pressing my hands over it, feeling how tight my clothes were, or lifting up my top and looking in the mirror to check how bloated I looked. I was extremely self-conscious at this time.

Straight after my Psychology degree I did a Ph.D. and had my first baby. I had my second child three years later, and only worked part-time in an academic position during this time. Symptoms actually remitted and I had a few years of complete relief. Life was relatively calm and stable as was my mood.

## CFS

In the year 2000, at the age of 33, I experienced a major life event. Having been adopted as a baby, I had the most loving parents and siblings and positive beliefs about being adopted. It wasn't until becoming a mother myself that I began to be curious about my biological background. With my parents' support I did a search and was reunited with many relatives. Initially this was an extremely positive experience, but over time some unexpected emotional reactions began to manifest. I basically had what I would describe as an identity crisis, almost like a shattering of my previous self, not knowing who I was or how to integrate the vast amount of new information I had learnt. I began to feel extremely tired all the time, couldn't concentrate or tolerate more than one sensory stimulus at a time, and had brain fog. My short-term memory was poor so I became forgetful and could not always think of the correct word to say in a sentence, often saying inappropriate words, or jumbled sentences, without even noticing. Having completed a Ph.D. only 4 years earlier, I couldn't even write a paragraph of text. My mood became very low and I had the IBS symptoms again. This time I became obsessed with trying to 'cure myself', so focused all my attention and energy on finding solutions and remedies to make my stomach feel better. I was ignoring (or avoiding) all the other more serious symptoms, believing that the IBS was 'the problem'.

I refused to see my GP for over a year, by which time my condition had deteriorated and I was only working one day a week, and not functioning well across all activities of daily living. This denial of recognising the problem, and pushing myself through, caused increased suffering which I felt even more responsible to resolve. The cycle was unrelenting and it took two years before I admitted that I needed help. In 2002 I was referred to an Immunology clinic where I was diagnosed with CFS. I received a course of individual CBT with a very skilled and experienced cognitive behavioural therapist. I still found it hard to recognise or accept that I was clinically depressed so engagement was initially difficult for me. I remember her patience and openness to try different methods with me as I found activity scheduling too demanding and not very engaging. On discovering my love of colour we devised a colour-coded version of the diary, like a traffic light system to denote how much fatigue each activity caused – green easiest, blue middle and red most demanding. This was a simple but effective adjustment that fitted my individual identity and increased my engagement in therapy. I was also introduced to the Mind over Mood (Greenberger & Padesky, 2015) and Coping with Chronic Fatigue Syndrome (Chalder, 1995) self-help guides, both of which I found helpful during this time.

It took another two years before I accepted any medication so the CBT alone only had limited benefit at the time, as clearly the biological symptoms were severe. To be honest, apart from the traffic light method, and the therapist's lovely compassionate manner, I remember very little of the therapy due to the cognitive deficits associated with CFS. The main impact this experience had, however, was that the therapist believed me and validated by distress, which made it easier for me to accept help. Eventually I went into remission and started to function better, but this probably took much longer due to my belief system to which we will now turn.

## Cognitive formulation

For the sake of this chapter, I shall provide a very simplified version of my formulation. I will begin with a Beckian longitudinal formulation as a possible explanation for the onset and development of my beliefs, and what may have made me vulnerable to developing these conditions, and once diagnosed prevented me from seeking help when I needed it.

This rule accounts for the self-reliance due to not being believed by doctors when a child, and being dismissed as 'nervous'. When there is a risk of being seen as 'nervous' then this activates the 'I am weak' core belief. This is why I found it hard to show emotions, as it risked being judged, which again would activate the 'I am weak' belief. By working hard in general, then this rule also serves to challenge the 'I am vulnerable' belief as it gives a sense of being strong. This emphasises how alluring this rule is, and how it drives the belief system to maintain unhealthy behaviours that increase the risk of adverse physical and mental health problems.

I experienced increased levels of hyperarousal symptoms, insomnia and fatigue. I became increasingly reliant on my rule – 'If I work hard enough, then I can achieve anything' in order to try and heal everyone else who I was treating in isolation from my team environment. This activated my positive core belief 'I am special' as this can make me believe I can achieve outcomes just by having the desire to want to help others. It is the belief that most healthcare professionals hold about wanting to change the world or make a difference, that can give rise to an almost 'superhuman' sense of self. I sometimes visualise myself as a superhero flying through the sky with cape and wand, wanting to save everyone. So when pushing myself made me feel physically and emotionally stressed I responded differently this time: I asked for help.

### Early experiences

- Very loving family life. Youngest of three children, all adopted as babies.
- Made to feel special (as I was 'chosen').
- I had chronic stomach ache from 5 years old and had anuresis until I was 7. Dismissed by GP as being a 'nervous' child.
- Referred to Paediatrician at 7 who did an X-ray and found an abnormality on my bladder. I had a total of two operations as first one was not successful. Recovered, but had recurrent UTIs as a teenager. I was on antibiotics for a number of years.
- Didn't show my emotions, so when upset would 'hold it in' (freeze response)
- Recurrent tonsilitis but not deemed frequent enough to warrant a referral for a tonsilectomy.
- On reflection I believe I had glandular fever as a teenager which went undiagnosed. This is important in terms of my autoimmune vulnerability to developing CFS, which was previously known as Myalgic Encephalomyelitis (ME).

### Core beliefs

**Positive core beliefs**
- I am loved
- I am special

**Negative core beliefs**
- I am vulnerable
- I am weak (emotionally – labelled as 'nervous child')
- Others are unreliable (doctors)

### Dominant Rule for living

If I work hard enough, then I can achieve anything – ALL OR NOTHING

### Critical incidents

When diagnosed with IBS although doctors did take this seriously I still tried to heal myself. The same was true on a larger and more detrimental level when I was diagnosed with CFS. I did not even ask for help for two years, resisting a diagnosis of depression as this reinforced my core belief that 'I am weak', triggering my all or nothing rule to try and cure myself without help.

## Recent critical incident

During the Covid-19 pandemic as a CBT therapist in a busy IAPT service, the stress of delivering CBT remotely for many months alone, from home, led to a chronic stress response. I believe I contracted the virus early on in the first wave in March 2020. I had to take two weeks off, and the post-viral recovery took several weeks or months. I experienced joint pain and muscle weakness for about 6-8 weeks, and used several splints and aids. I continued working as these symptoms gradually declined, but general stress of working with mounting levels of distress in my patients caused other difficulties.

## Functional analysis of my stress reaction

In an attempt to try and respond differently to stress during this recent episode, I decided to take a different approach. As helpful as it is to understand the activation of the belief system it does not necessarily lead to change with regard to the rule. I needed a different way of conceptualising it, so turned to Learning Theory and behaviourism.

Ferster (1973) provides an eloquent account of a functional analysis of depression, which draws on Skinner's original work on operant conditioning. The writings in the book 'Science and Human Behaviour' (Skinner, 1955) resonated at a personal level. I started to see how a functional analysis could help me focus on the behaviours that maintain my resistance to seeking help.

The first example shows how 'getting through' stressful periods in the past became the conditioned response to stress triggers, regardless of how bad the physical and emotional symptoms were. I needed to break this association by changing the behaviour, so in my recent example I asked for help when the symptoms became noticeable and had a negative impact – couldn't relax or sleep, little energy for family activities, lower mood. These are my early warning signs and need to be seen as triggers in a functional analysis sense. Triggers to a relapse in my physical and mental health. Asking for help and taking a complete break from work was VERY HARD to do, as it felt so unnatural and dangerous. This is due to the fear response that had become associated with asking for help right back from

Table 10.1 Me in the past

| Antecedents | Behaviour | Consequences |
| --- | --- | --- |
| Stress | Push on, often using unhelpful coping strategies such as working longer hours to try and get everything done, and using alcohol | Physical and emotional demise BUT got through it without seeking help. |

*Table 10.2* Me during this recent episode of work-related stress

| Antecedents | Behaviour | Consequences |
| --- | --- | --- |
| Stress | Rang in sick and asked for help. Had two weeks off on sick leave. | Recovered within two weeks and returned to work. No one treated me any differently. In fact, I felt cared for. |

being a little girl – if I ask for help I won't be believed and will be seen as being 'emotional' or 'nervous'. Pushing through and trying to heal myself felt like a less threatening action, but over time served to reinforce the negative effects of not asking for help. A key factor was that my line manager said 'Helen, I believe you', which was critical to allowing myself to be helped. It was as if she was giving me permission to stop working and rest. It was a very compassionate approach and it worked for me. My recovery was much quicker this time and I did not have the same level of negative emotional response to being off sick as I have in the past – such as shame, guilt and anxiety.

## The role of mindfulness and self-compassion

I am aware that attentional focus and self-critical thinking have been significant factors in maintaining my stress reactions and management. I have been hyper-alert to physical symptoms such as abdominal bloating, insomnia and fatigue which give rise to increased worry, rumination and catastrophic thinking. In order to break this cycle, I have been practicing mindfulness for the past 7 years. During the pandemic and lock down period I focused more on present-moment experience by increasing my mindfulness practices. I would use meditation and go for mindful walks daily, paying more attention to sensory information 'outside my head' to keep me grounded. Recognising the role alcohol has played in stress management in the past – to reward myself for 'working hard', or as a coping strategy to manage symptoms – I decided to take a complete break from drinking alcohol for several months. This reinforced my learning that I CAN manage stress without using alcohol or any other means for self-soothing.

Self-compassion is incredibly challenging for healthcare professionals. This is related to a dysfunctional belief that helping others requires putting their needs before our own. This leads to a set of behaviours that serve to neglect our own needs at every level. An example I often use is this scenario – imagine you are listening to a patient telling you something, and it is the end of the allotted session time. This story they are telling you is very detailed and possibly not significant or important in terms of their treatment, but rather than attend to your physical need to end the session you put your patient's emotional need first. It sounds like a simple example but when multiplied across different situations over time the impact becomes exponential.

I started to practise what I guided patients to do, and in 2018 completed a work book on self-compassion with my colleague and supervisor who was also a cognitive behavioural therapist. We set ourself this challenge and it was life changing. We learned so much from observing our self-critical thoughts and associated actions. An example was waking up later than normal for work as I had hit the 'snooze' button three times. In the past I would have been angry with myself saying things like 'you idiot, you should have got up straight away, now you're going to be late, and you'll let people down' leading to the threat response of anxiety and fear of negative appraisal and outcomes. I would normally negate my need for breakfast or coffee and rush to work. However, when I had started responding in a more compassionate way this is what actually happened when I overslept. On waking, I calculated that I could still get there 20 minutes before my first patient appointment was due. Instead of jumping out of bed and rushing to work angry and anxious, I decided to still have a quick shower, eat breakfast and make a fresh coffee, as I could still arrive before the first appointment. And what a difference this made. I felt the positive effects of this self-care act by not feeling angry, guilty or anxious, which reduced worry and rumination and self-critical thoughts, and I arrived at work in a calm state – despite over-sleeping!

I continue to practise self-compassion and mindfulness for my own relapse prevention and general well-being. It has also helped me to empathise and understand what challenges my patients face when asked to do any of the CBT interventions described in this book. From the account I have presented in this chapter, I have clearly tried pretty much all interventions on myself and this insight has so many benefits for my own practice when working with this client group. Acknowledging suffering, and difficulties asking for help, have been beneficial when trying to engage someone who is presenting with characteristics in common with my own lived experience.

In summary, I have presented a brief overview of some of the factors that have contributed to my own difficulties living with long-term and medically-unexplained symptoms which are both triggered by stress. I have attempted to demonstrate how using a broad CBT framework has helped me to understand the onset, development and maintenance of problems associated with CFS and IBS, and apply interventions from each wave of CBT to maintain my recovery and prevent relapse. In your own practice you may come across people with similar experiences, and it is likely that if they are asking for help it has taken a very long time to get to you. In fact, remember, that by asking for help they are likely breaking one of their rules, which we know is distressing. The take home messages I would like to leave are; to validate the person's suffering, giving them permission to be helped, and to be open and flexible in your use of CBT interventions and techniques. Also, you can normalise their presentation, and even share this chapter with them, to show that others struggle in the same way (even therapists). If standard approaches do not seem to be working, try more creative methods to engage and empower the person. Once equipped with a greater understanding of the formulation and a set of tools to use, you will have helped that person much more than you may realise, as results may occur years down the line as they did for me. Be aware of your own rules for living that may cause you the same kinds of problems as the person with LTC or MUS – pushing yourself to rescue or cure – whereas acceptance of your own role in the process will manage your expectations.

# Chapter 11

# Ways of helping MUS patients to change negative behaviours

It is important to understand why patients with MUS alter their behaviours, and why this may contribute to their symptoms. This change may be related to idiosyncratic cognitions, or to bodily sensations such as chronic pain or fatigue. To take a simple example like pain; after the patient has experienced debilitating pain, possibly in response to a sensitisation process, he may then develop distressing cognitions such as 'this pain will damage me', or 'this pain will not stop', or 'this pain will be unbearable'. This will then invoke an emotion of fear, which will then drive avoidance behaviour. The consequences of this avoidance are that the person may experience deconditioning, which will intensify the pain experience further. The other consequence is that the person may fail to learn that his thoughts are distorted or unhelpful. We can say with confidence that if the patient is fearful that then he will exaggerate the threat and downplay his ability to cope (to a greater or lesser extent), as this is what anxiety theory suggests (Beck, Emery & Greenberg, 2005). Avoidance may generalise to work and social activities, and relationships, which may worsen the person's mood, and make the pain harder to bear. A similar thing may happen in chronic fatigue where the individual worries that his fatigue may significantly deteriorate if he exercises or exerts himself. In irritable bowel, the avoidance is mainly driven by a fear of being incontinent, or of passing wind in public, or having embarrassing bowel symptoms. It may partly be driven by patients experiencing discomfort and pain and not wanting to be out and doing activities whilst suffering these symptoms. In non-epileptic seizures, the avoidance may be related to an automatic or deliberate avoidance of stress, or trauma related memories. The patient may also behaviourally avoid triggers, if they can identify what these are. They may also avoid living a more normal life because of fears of being injured if they have a seizure outside. With the non-epileptic seizures there is some actual danger, particularly in situations such as using dangerous machinery, crossing roads, or bathing, but often the person's level of avoidance is disproportionate to the risk.

Other patterns that have been noticed are boom and bust, otherwise known as activity fluctuation: this is where a person may avoid tasks because of the effects of fatigue, will then have a burst of energy which encourages them to engage in excessive activity. The consequence of this is that the person will then worsen

DOI: 10.4324/9780367824433-15

their fatigue symptoms. The excessive activity may be driven by perfectionist rules, so, the person may push themselves to be busy and to engage in excessive activity, they are following the demands of the rule. When they crash out, they are unable to follow these demands, and are likely to engage in self-critical talk, which may worsen their mood. The consequences of this pattern are that the person poorly manages their lifestyle and activities. There can be patterns of avoidance in all medically unexplained symptoms, and it is important to assess the idiosyncratic cognition that drives these.

Safety behaviours occur when the person perceives something as being dangerous, and this is not actually the case. From a cognitive therapy perspective, the function of the safety behaviour is to minimise or avoid the risk from the trigger. In learning theory, safety seeking behaviours are viewed as getting in the way of natural habituation to a trigger. These safety behaviours will commonly occur in chronic pain where there is such a fear of the pain, that the person may guard himself by adopting an unusual posture, by doing activities in an unusual way such as very slowly, or by taking excessive medication, and a similar process occurs in chronic fatigue. In IBS type presentations the person, if they are over worried about the risk of being incontinent, may restrict what they eat, monitor where all the toilets are, only eat at home, carry incontinence pads around with them, etc. When health anxiety is part of the picture, the individual may poke and prod their body, check their pulse and blood pressure and appearance, take inappropriate medication and seek excessive reassurance from the GP, from relatives and from the Internet.

There may be a more general category of behaviours in this group, in which patients will do things for idiosyncratic reasons related to the symptoms they have, or the illness they are concerned about, and this may be problematic. This may include becoming over reliant on others, giving up work, becoming preoccupied with their condition, spending a lot of time investigating their condition, using alternative medicine, eating a strange diet, etc.

**Understanding behaviours**

Questions to ask to understand these behaviours are:

- Do you feel you could manage your symptoms better? Do you relatives think you cope with your symptoms well? What do you think your GP would say about how you are manging your symptoms?
- Do you avoid anything because you're worried about your symptoms? Is there anywhere you would not go? Is there anything you would not do?
- Do you make the best use of health advice?
- Do you seek excessive reassurance because you're worried? Is this from the Internet, your GP, your relatives, or from anywhere else?
- Do you avoid anything because of your symptoms?
- Do you do anything extra to manage your symptoms? It's what you are doing extra, helpful? Is what you were doing extra causing you any problems?
- Have you changed your eating pattern? Have you changed your exercise pattern?

It is important to engage in dialogue with the patient to understand why they are doing these things, to make a judgement together as to whether they are helpful (to their health, well-being and valued goals), particularly in the medium and longer term, and what alternative behaviours may be better. This is done in the spirit of guided discovery, and collaboration. Typical reasons patients engage in these behaviours are: to make their symptoms better or to prevent them getting worse, or to clear them up completely; to reassure themselves that their symptoms are not dangerous; to minimise or eliminate pain or fatigue feelings; to help them understand the symptoms with the hope of getting a solution.

Sometimes it is difficult to work out whether the person's behaviour is constructive or unhelpful, examples of this uncertainty could be going back to work, remaining on sickness benefits, pursuing experimental treatments, taking certain medications, engaging in unusual alternative treatments, etc. As therapists we will approach this by asking questions such as is this behaviour rational, does it follow scientific guidelines and evidence, could it lead to physical or financial harm, does it serve the medium- to long-term valued interests of the patient? These questions should be borne in mind when the therapist is engaging in a dialogue with the patient around these behaviours.

When we are discussing these behaviours, we would help the patient think about the following:

- Avoidant behaviours are problematic for several reasons: they can lead to the process of deconditioning, where the person's muscles, because they are not used, become more easily painful or fatigued. They are also problematic because they stop the person challenging exaggerated thoughts such as 'I will be harmed if I do this' or 'the symptoms will be intolerable', or 'I will soil myself or wet myself'. Also, because they stop the person living a full and valued life, and meeting their personal goals.
- Safety behaviours are problematic for similar reasons; they stop the person learning that their thoughts may be exaggerated. They can also worsen the actual symptom, an example of this is where the health anxious person prods the stomach, or rubs the skin, and worsens the existing symptom.
- Both safety and avoidant behaviours are problematic, in the sense that if the person does get some short-term relief from an avoidant, safety, or escape behaviour, then this behaviour will be negatively re-enforced and will become the automatic behaviour of choice, often out of the person's awareness.

There are some questions that can be asked to help the therapist address the unhelpful behaviours: 'I'm aware that you engage in a lot of avoiding behaviours or safety or other behaviours because of your pain/symptoms. I just wondered why you do these? What would go through your mind if you stop doing them? What are the shorter and longer-term consequences of being avoidant? Is it more important to get shorter term relief from your symptoms, or to do the things you truly value in your life? If you do your activities and your symptoms flare-up is there any better ways of coping with this at the time? Could we change something about your thinking, your attention, your emotions, your behaviour? Is it possible to carry the symptoms with you whilst you are fully engaged in the activity you really want to do?'

Here are two clinical examples, Jim and Margaret, to illustrate the aforementioned points:

Jim is a retired academic who suffers from depression and chronic pain. His negative behaviours are:

- Taking a lot of opiate analgesia (understandably to reduce the severity of the pain, but with a negative effect of drowsiness and habituation to the dose);
- Withdrawing from interacting with his wife (related to negative thoughts that she does not want to see him, he has nothing to offer, he won't get on with her family and he will be asked to do activities that will worsen the pain).
- Spending quite a lot of time trying to find a solution to the pain (related to a belief that all problems can be solved).
- Ruminating on why he has ended up like this (to try to discover a solution).
- Adopting a tense, guarded posture (to brace himself against someone bumping into him).
- Disengaging from professional activities (because he does not feel he has anything to offer, and that he would not be able to cope with the demands of travel).

Margaret frequently has non – epileptic seizures. She was collapsing 6–10 times weekly, and this was impacting on her life. Initially it was hard to see what may be causing these, on assessment they seemed to be triggered by stress when she had to interact with her ex-husband, or she had a flashback to past traumas. She used to be often beaten by her husband in a pub that they ran whilst the children were nearby in the house, and as she could not escape, she could only freeze.

Her current behaviour is to avoid all memories of the trauma by:

- Not talking about it
- Not seeing her ex-husband
- Not going to the location where it happened
- Downplaying the importance of the trauma (these behaviours are to avoid the anxiety, the sense of being threatened, it happening again, and the potential for a seizure)

## Changing behaviours

There are a number of ways to help patients reduce unhelpful behaviours. These would include: behavioural experiments, activity scheduling, working towards goals and problem solving.

Behavioural experiments are based on ideas from cognitive therapy: they can test the patient's existing beliefs about themselves, others, or the world; they can construct and test new, more adaptive beliefs; they can contribute to the development and verification of the formulation (Bennett-Levy et al., 2004). There are two designs of experiments the first one is *hypothesis testing* experiments, which are usually testing out the truth or helpfulness of a particular thought, for example 'if I told people about my irritable bowel, they would reject me, and I couldn't stand it.' Or, 'if I don't keep monitoring my symptoms, I'm going to miss an occurrence of cancer.' Or, 'I need to find a medical explanation for my symptoms before I can live a normal life.' The other type of experiment is *discovery experiments* when patients have little or no idea about the process of what is maintaining a problem, or what may happen if they act in a different way (Bennett-Levy et al., 2004): an example is 'I will ask people like me who have pain, what their experience of exercise is'. There are also two designs of experiments the first one being *active experiments*, which are most common, patients will do something different and see what happens and reflect on the truth of their perception. The second design is *observational experiments* where the person simply observes the situation, without altering it, and tries to learn from it.

A behavioural experiment is structured using a behavioural experiment form, which are freely available on the internet, and on excellent specialist sites such as Psychology Tools. One would write the negative thought and associated thoughts to be tested, at the top of the form, (it is a good idea to write several thoughts/ hypotheses down, as if one is not confirmed as expected, there are others to learn from: this principle of a 'no lose experiment' is a good one to use with this group, and in general). The strength of belief in the thought is rated (this should be measured as if the person is about to do the experiment). The alternative thought is worked out with the patient, and the strength of belief is rated as the person imagines just being about to do it. The experiment is planned, and then executed in the session, or outside. Often experiments are best started in the therapy sessions, especially if there is any danger of the person being injured or suffering undue pain. After the experiment(s) the patient is asked to fill in the back of the sheet noting what he observed and how this related to the target cognition. He will also reflect on what he can do to test out the cognition further. Often the person will gain some helpful information, but there needs to be a considerable amount of repetition to strengthen the belief. Examples of BE's are: the patient is reluctant to ask for help, associated with thought such as, 'If I ask for help, I will be rejected', an active experiment here would be to ask for help, perhaps from a person that they felt there is some chance of responding positively. An observational experiment is to observe instances of where other people ask for help and how the other person responds. When the BE is being planned a lot of attention needs to go in to any problems the person will have doing it, observing it and reflecting on it, but more particularly the first of these. Often the obstacle is the person's belief that their fearful thoughts are true. One can address this by referring to any cognitive restructuring that has already been done, where the evidence for and against the truthfulness of the belief is tested. One can also grade it, asking the person to do something at an easier level. One should do what one can to minimise the risk of any actual danger to the patient, for example from falling, as described in the following example.

This patient has functional neurological symptoms and has difficulty walking, and tends to walk holding on to the wall. Their cognitions are 'I won't be able to balance if I don't hold on', belief 80%, 'If I can't balance, I will fall', belief 70%', 'If I fall, I will seriously injure myself', belief 50%', 'If I fall, I won't be able to get up', belief 50%, 'If I fall, no one will help me', belief 60%. Thinking about any risks in this experiment, the patient may have had a history of falls, and understandably may be frightened of these. Here we could start off with something that may be less challenging such as the person worrying, they would not be able to get up from a fall, and we would test out that thought. One could have a detailed discussion with the patient about ways to get up from the ground, any adaptions she would have to make to this. When she sat on the ground and tried this, I (PK) would stand beside her, encouraging her, I would be ready to help if necessary. To do something like this one would have to have confidence that the patient is able to do it. It may be helpful to get a physiotherapist involved, if this is possible, or to do the walk in a carpeted area. If the person has significant deconditioning or a muscle wasting, then it may be necessary for the person to practise muscle strengthening exercises, prescribed by the physiotherapist. There are a set of exercises tailored to chronic fatigue patients available on our website Fatiguefighter. org.uk developed by Philip and his physiotherapist colleague Anne Childs.

As stated previously patients with MUS do not usually have the typical pattern of health anxiety such as worrying that they have fatal illness: if they do the approach would be as described in Chapter 6. The health anxious thoughts tend to be around the impact of the symptoms, conviction that they have an illness that will continue and impact on their lives; the behaviours that can come from this are: avoidance of getting on with normal life activities, spending time looking for a cure of the illness.

Activity scheduling, as a behavioural change, is where first of all, a record is made of the person's hour by hour activity. An analysis is made of this, to try to decide how patterns of activity are contributing to problems. There is then an attempt to help the person schedule a different pattern of activity that is more helpful. This can be quite complex in terms of considering what the person should note in their diary, how to interpret the diary when it is returned, and how to plan the behavioural change. So, in planning the diary a classic way of doing this would be to get the person to write down what they are doing on an hourly basis, and to rate themselves on measures of mastery and pleasure, this being particularly helpful if someone is depressed. An alternative way of doing this is to keep an hour-by-hour diary and to rate the severity of the target symptom, this task will be cognitively demanding, and the patient may benefit from the creative methods, such as colour coding, described in Chapters 7 and 9. A generic diary for doing this is provided in Chapter 2. The diary could combine a description of daily activities, with a rating of emotion and a rating of symptoms. When choosing the format of the diary, it is good for the therapist to consider what type of information they would like to gather, and this can be done collaboratively with the patient, for example one could ask 'if we were going to record what you were doing each day, what is it about your symptoms mood or behaviour that we should try and capture?' In the therapist's mind, this may be triggers for symptoms (and the triggers may be quite immediate or may be more diffuse), it may be the relationship between the activity, emotion and the symptom.

It is important that the patient is on board with keeping a detailed diary, and any hesitation or doubt should be addressed. When the diary is returned there is an artistry in analysing the information. Things to bear in mind are

- General patterns such as avoidance and withdrawal: in the diary there may be a lot of entries around being in bed, getting up late, not going out, being away from people, solitary activities, watching TV. Physical symptoms such as pain and fatigue may be rated low (in the sense of not being too bad) during this, as may mastery and pleasure scores, but mood may be worse.
- Specific patterns of avoidance, for example, of walking, eating certain foods, taking exercise, going to the GP, interacting with family, attending appointments at the hospital.
- Boom and bust pattern, what is observed is the patient doing a lot of activities at once, or one after the other, with little rest or break. On following days there can be a pattern of inactivity or avoidance in response to a flair up of symptoms which may be rated as severe.
- Overdoing it: the pattern may be one of the patient being continually active, doing lots of activities, particularly doing lots for other people. This pattern of behaviour may reflect underlying rules around perfectionism and self-sacrifice. Patient scores on physical symptoms will likely demonstrate severity.

Example: it was clear that Kirsten was very anxious about activity. She had been spending prolonged periods in bed, looked anxious and identified thoughts such as, 'If I'm more active I'll definitely get worse, and I could cause injury to myself. The pain will be unbearable.' She was anxious and avoidant. She predicted that her pain would be a ten out of ten. We spent a long time on the therapeutic relationship, the idea that 'hurt does not equal harm', and the concept of deconditioning. She started off spending short periods out of bed, then short periods (five to ten minutes) standing, then taking a few steps, then increasing her steps. After three months she can walk a few hundred yards with tolerable pain, and treatment is ongoing. She rates her pain at seven, and she is challenging previous attributions.

## Physical exercise in MUS

Activity and exercise are across the board good, abundant scientific evidence has demonstrated that physically active people of all age groups and ethnicities have higher levels of cardiorespiratory fitness, health and wellness, and a lower risk for developing several chronic medical illnesses, including cardiovascular disease, compared with those who are physically inactive. Although more intense and longer durations of physical activity correlate directly with improved outcomes, even small amounts of physical activity provide protective health benefits (Fletcher et al., 2018). However, looking at MUS, a study from 2002 showed that aerobic exercise was not superior to a control group of stretching, but the incidence of attending GP and obtaining prescriptions was reduced (Peters, Stanley, Rose, Kaney & Salmon, 2002). Evidence of fair methodological quality suggests that walking is associated with significant improvements in outcome compared with a control intervention in chronic musculoskeletal pain conditions, but longer-term effectiveness is uncertain. Walking can be recommended as an effective form of exercise or activity for individuals with chronic musculoskeletal pain but should be supplemented with strategies aimed at maintaining participation. (O'Connor et al., 2015). Sometimes patients are fearful of exercising worrying that it may damage them, escalate the symptoms, or cause intolerable pain. This is best addressed through open dialogue about the risks of this, and behavioural experiments starting at a lower level of exercise

## Problem Solving

This strategy, which was briefly discussed in Chapter 4, involves helping patients address difficult and stressful situations which could include dealing with a physical illness, a financial crisis, having to move home or dealing with a deteriorating personal relationship. It is known that there are more stressful life events at the onset of MUS, particularly chronic fatigue syndrome and as stated the stress arising from these problems may be a maintenance factor in MUS: this is more a clinical impression, than an evidence-based conclusion. There is evidence that this approach can be used effectively as a sole therapy with depression, and indeed helping cancer patients cope (D'Zurilla & Nezu, 2010). If it is used then there is a well-established protocol (Neenan & Dryden, 2013).

1   Problem Identification. It is important here to define the problem in precise language, for example 'I am likely to be made redundant in March, because of my health problems, which will lead to a 75% reduction of my income'
2   Goal Selection. Again, the person should express this clearly and in a way that is measurable.
3   Generation of alternatives. This step is to generate as many workable solutions as possible, even if they are highly unlikely (often called 'brainstorming'). Sometimes the therapist needs to prompt the person to get them started.
4   Consideration of consequences. The next stage is to consider the advantages and disadvantages of each alternative. If one wanted to elaborate then one could consider this in the short and long-term and even the consequences for significant other people.

5    Decision-making. Here the person is asked to consider the alternatives that help them reach their goals. There may be one or more. This is the most difficult stage, as one can be faced with several possibilities that look equally attractive, or more often unattractive. It may help to give a numerical value to each alternative on a scale of 1–10. This could measure 'usefulness' or 'desirableness.' It is probably necessary at this stage to have quite a prolonged discussion with the patient and they are likely to require time to think about it and discuss it with friends/family. It is important that one does not impose one's preferred solution onto the patient, though that can be tempting.

6    Implementation. If the person has made up their mind then the next stage is to put it into practice. Depending on the task, this may be difficult. As before, role-play, grading and discussion of the consequences are the things to do.

7    Evaluation. Did the implementing of the solution achieve the goal, or move them towards the goal? If it did not, it may be the person has implemented the solution inadequately or without persistence, or they are lacking in the necessary skills to do so. It may also be that there are real life obstacles to achieving it. If the desired goal is not achieved, one might work with further coaching in the skills to help achieve the solution or the person may have to return to considering rejected alternatives.

### An example of problem solving with MUS

Janie describes her main problem as feeling tired and weak in her legs, with strange sensations and she occasionally feels dizzy. She believes she cannot do as much as she used to do, or her muscles get more painful. She worried a bit in the past that she had multiple sclerosis but does now accept that it is not that. She worries that if she pushes on, she will have to sit down and be 'stuck' somewhere. She feels the problems are essentially stress related, the onset the previous year, after she started in a new job in clinical trials as a statistician. Her first trial went wrong and this was stressful, she had lots of responsibility and was working long days. One of her managers at work was difficult and set unrealistic targets for the work. This first therapy task here was to develop a formulation, and it was not too difficult. The factors identified were: she was under considerable stress from the demands of work and this was contributing to tiredness and weakness. She would avoid exercising, and took excessive rest, which was contributing to deconditioning. Part of treatment was to teach problem solving as follows:

T: it looks like we agree on some of the things that are contributing to your symptoms. As part of your CBT, I would like to teach you a technique called problem-solving, and we can use it to address these problems. (therapist explains the stages of problem-solving identified earlier: problem identification, goal selection, generation of alternatives, consideration of consequences, decision-making, implementation and evaluation).

P: OK, I am happy with this problem statement, 'I have too many unrealistic targets at work, set by a manager. I often stay late at work to try to achieve the goals. This stress and overwork contribute to my symptoms. I have no time to exercise which used to help me.'

We discussed a goal which was 'I will reduce my current targets in half. I will only stay late twice a week. I will exercise for 45 minutes, twice a week'. We went through different options and generated some actions: speaking to her manager; enrolling in the gym, working from home one day, asking colleagues to help more, the first of these being most important. She did speak to him with some trepidation, and this helped them both understand the demands on them, her work was reorganised to a degree, another person was organised to help with some of the workload, it was not expected that she would always stay late. This was implemented and although not everything she wanted happened, the solution did allow her to work less, be less concerned about targets, and to fit in exercise, and this did lead to a reduction in symptoms.

## Helping patients take gradual behavioural steps towards goals

There are a number of principles here that should be followed. During assessment, the patient should be asked in general terms about what they want to gain from therapy, and what their goals are. When they come into therapy, more formal problem and targets should be done. The patient's SMART goals should be written down: smart goals are, specific, manageable, achievable, realistic and time-limited. The smart goals should always be in the patient and therapist's mind as they undergo therapy, and there should always be a momentum towards them. Here are some examples of smart goals with MUS patients.

- By the end of therapy, I will be back at work and I will tolerate my pain for 30 minutes before I consider pain relief.
- I will understand the maintenance factors that contribute to my fatigue.
- In three months, I will be able to swim 6 lengths in the pool.
- In three months, my irritable bowel symptoms will be at a level in which I am able to go to the gym for one hour twice weekly
- I will not have any non-epileptic seizures
- I will independently go to the shops, without using safety behaviours, twice weekly
- My pain will reduce to a level that will allow me to do a 30-minute walk twice daily.

## Medication management

Sometimes it feels that patients mismanage their prescribed medication use, and this is contributing for example to fatigue. This could be either not taking medications that can be helpful (often because they think they should be able to cope without it), taking excessive medications, not having medication reviewed on a regular basis or taking the wrong type of medication for the problem. It could be argued that it is not the responsibility of the cognitive behavioural therapist to interfere with this process, however this often comes up as an issue. When it is obvious that medication is a problem, the first thing is to explore this Socratically, 'when did you last have your medication reviewed?', 'do you think you've got your medication right?', 'do you think your medication could be contributing to your symptoms in some way?', 'Do you understand what your medications are for?', 'are you taking your medication as prescribed?' etc. Sometimes the patient can have a very constructive conversation with you about this, other times they just don't know. Some drugs are very sedating, some cause odd side effects, some are addictive. Depending what comes out of the conversation, it will be useful to involve the GP in trying to get the patient's medication exactly right. Possible strategies are getting the medication reviewed, tracking symptoms and medication use links, educating the patient about the effects of each medication, addressing reservations about taking certain medications, dealing with addictions to medications, helping the patient to take the medication at the right time and at the right dose, and helping the patient take the minimum amount of medication that they need.

## Reassurance

In health anxiety, as an anxiety disorder, there is a considerable problem with reassuring seeking, and this may also be the case in medically unexplained symptoms where patients are over-anxious about the cause and consequences of their symptoms. So, in medically unexplained symptoms, with symptoms like pain, fatigue, headaches, constipation and seizures there is likely to be a greater or lesser degree of reassurance seeking. Reassurance is looked for because the person has a symptom they are worried about, and there may be an intolerance of uncertainty. They are looking for a relative, or a doctor, or the Internet to tell them that they have nothing to worry about, but unfortunately it does not work. They are likely to be given contradictory information if they look for reassurance from different people, or the same person in different times, and this can increase a sense of uncertainty. A doctor may offer them further investigations, possibly willingly, or sometimes under duress. The period they wait to get these investigations can be a period of great anxiety, culminating in relief when they are told that nothing can be found. If the reassuring successfully reduces anxiety, then the person will get some relief from this, and the behaviour will become negatively reinforced and will continue. Another problem can be that if the person has an anxious state, there is more focus on more threatening parts of the information, particularly from the GP or from the Internet. The GP may say 'it's nothing to worry about, but I'll send you for tests just in case', the patient will focus on the phrase 'just in case.'

How to present the rationale for reducing unhelpful reassurance: 'Because you are worried about the symptom you are seeking reassurance . . . what do you think of that idea . . . let me understand why you are doing it . . . What thoughts would come up for you if you stopped?',' Are you willing to stop this, or at least reduce it?', 'Let's fill a behavioural experiment sheet in and test out your worries'. The typical worries that come up when the person stops reassurance are: that they may have cancer and this will be quickly getting worse; that they need to get a diagnosis straight away and start treatment; that the symptom will get significantly worse quite quickly; that if left untreated, they could die soon.

## Sleep related behaviours

For the patient who sleeps too much again it is important to assess why this is occurring. Is the patient trying to escape something through sleep? Is the excessive sleep (over the standard eight hours) causing problems? Even if the patient is saying that it isn't causing problems, it is normally considered a problem because excessive time in bed could breed further inactivity and may contribute to deconditioning, also excessive daytime sleep may affect the person's ability to sleep at night. It is a matter of judgement as to whether one should try to reduce this because the person may be catching up after a period of significant exhaustion. There may be a significant difference between the person who for a few weeks is taking nine to ten hours to catch up, and the person who for months has been sleeping very excessively, the latter being problematic. If one is going to help the person reduce to, say, eight hours, then the most important thing is to do it gradually: for example, the person could reduce 15 minutes each week and clinical experience would suggest that most patients could successfully do this. Experience would also suggest that if sleep can be improved then this can have an impact on symptoms, particularly fatigue symptoms.

A problem that is difficult to solve is the patient with chronic pain who struggles to sleep because of the pain. The presence of sleep disturbances and the number of health complaints predicted onset, persistence and worsening of pain and elimination of sleep problems in an early phase is an interesting approach in treating chronic pain. More research is needed to illuminate the possible pathogenetic relations between pain, non-specific health complaints, sleep problems and depression (Nitter, Pripp & Forseth, 2012). In another study sleep complaints were reported by 88% of the sample of 55 chronic pain patients. Pre-sleep cognitive arousal, rather than pain severity, was found to be the primary predictor of sleep quality. (Morin, Gibson & Wade, 1998) These authors also found that a standard behavioural approach to sleep worked well with pain patients. Currie, Wilson and Curran (2002) found that CBT could be effective for sleep, but only 18% were fully recovered from their sleep problems and patients improved more of they had lower sleep efficacy at baseline. In another study negative mood mediated the relationship between poor sleep and pain in a sample of 292 facial, back and fibromyalgia chronic pain patients (O'Brien et al., 2010). Some patients are given medications to help sleep and pain, these would include, antidepressants, antipsychotics, opioids and benzodiazepines. Patients may take over-the-counter analgesics such as paracetamol or ibuprofen (Cheatle et al., 2016). A large recent review showed pregabalin to be the most effective medication (Husak & Blair, 2020) There does not seem to be any data on the combination of CBT and medication.

## Health promotion model and behaviours

The health promotion model aims to prevent common physical health problems in the general population. Informed by public health and epidemiology, health promotion focuses on improving health (Green, Tones, Cross & Woodall, 2015). Four main health behaviours, which impact on mortality and quality of life, are targeted: nutrition, physical activity, smoking and alcohol use (Riekert, Ockene and Pbert, 2013). There is a requirement for conformity to the advice and recommended behaviour changes, and therefore health promotion is thwart with difficulties. Prochaska and DiClemente (1983) proposed the 'stages of change' model, outlining five stages a person needs to go through for effective behavioural change to occur. Relapse is an extra component that is commonly experienced with behavioural change. The stages are:

*   Pre-contemplation – this is the stage before the person has even thought about changing their behaviour. They may not even be aware of the risks of their behaviour at this stage. If they are, they may not want to change or play down the risks.
*   Contemplation – this is the stage where the person is considering making a change
*   Preparation – preparing for the change, planning how they will do it and when
*   Action – active change begins
*   Maintenance – this is the challenge of maintaining the change
*   Relapse – this can occur at any time during the action phase or when the new behaviour has been maintained over time. Once relapse occurs, the person may go back to the pre-contemplation stage or continue taking action to maintain the gains

How can we apply this to people with LTC and MUS? At the point of seeking psychological support, they may at any of these stages of change. Possibly they have tried to modify their behaviour previously and are now in the relapse phase, or have never considered that behavioural change could help their symptoms. It is our job, as the cognitive behavioural therapist, to motivate the person without being directive or patronising. The four targeted health promotion issues, listed earlier, are all likely to affect the maintenance of psychological distress associated with LTC. A knowledge of diet, exercise, modifying behaviours such as alcohol use and smoking is essential from the assessment, and these can be suggested as suitable goals for therapy.

## Chapter summary

Patients with these conditions can engage in unhelpful behaviours such as avoidance, or safety behaviours, reassurance, or poor problem-solving. The behaviours can arise from idiosyncratic cognitions, or more directly from experience of symptoms. Standard questions are asked to understand the functions of the behaviours then therapists can help patients problem-solving better, face situations, manage medications better and sleep better.

## Chapter 12

# Skills in working with cognition

In this chapter we will build on the formulation driven approach proposed by Deary et al. (2007) presented in Chapter 8, focusing on the different levels of cognition within the model. In particular, working at the rule and core belief levels will be explored in more detail, as these tend to be extremely rigid in patients with MUS. We also need to be mindful that working at a cognitive level is challenging due to the very nature of many of the MUS which make thinking, concentration and attentional focus compromised. CBT treatment is likely to take longer and require some adaptations and flexibility. We also emphasise that there is a lack of research evidence that working at this level is any more effective than the other interventions presented in the other chapters. However, both authors believe that, given sufficient time, expertise and strong therapeutic relationship, collaborative work at this level can produce some positive gains beyond initial symptom relief.

We will begin with a brief description of the three levels of cognition as defined by Beck in his original cognitive therapy theory, distinguishing between *content* (of the thoughts) and thinking *processes*. Some of the material here is covered in earlier chapters, as many of the issues outlined apply to both LTC and MUS. However, this chapter focuses more on how we can work at a cognitive level with patients with MUS and examples from both authors are presented.

## Negative automatic thoughts in MUS

Typically, in CBT, we consider three levels of thinking, namely thoughts (NATS), rules, and beliefs.

Regarding *thought content:* in Beck's model (1976) NATS are defined as an individual's appraisal of a specific situation or event (or symptom). As such this level of cognition represents what is going through an individual's mind in a particular situation, and may be associated with positive or negative emotions. The NATS that the clinician is most interested in are those that are most strongly associated with elevated levels of negative feelings such as anxiety, low mood, guilt, shame and anger and the like. NATS can occur in two forms: with content these can be words, or images. Each disorder specific CBT model identifies different themes in terms of the content of NATS (and rules for living). Thus, for example

DOI: 10.4324/9780367824433-16

in pain the content theme in NATS is a threatening misinterpretation of bodily sensations, where danger is imminent, typical NATS are, for example 'The pain will be unbearable', or 'I'm going to damage my body if I move', the second type of content is images, for example, the image of being paralysed, and people standing over you staring at you and not helping.

We need to intervene at this level when the cognition is contributing to the maintenance of the MUS. Examples of possible unhelpful thoughts are:

• 'I'm going to make my symptoms worse'
• 'I'm going to injure myself'
• 'I won't be able to cope with this symptom'
• 'Because I am ill people won't want to be with me'
• 'I might wet myself or soil myself'
• 'I'll have a seizure'

If the thought seems obviously distorted or unrealistic it can be approached by using the standard negative automatic thoughts diary technique. This would involve the patient keeping a diary of his thoughts every time his emotion changed, or he had a flareup of his symptoms. In the usual fashion, the person would look at evidence why the thought may be true, then, what is another way of thinking about it, why the thought may not be 100% true all of the time, what would they say to their best friend who had this thought, and finally, what is a more balanced thought. The patient would then be encouraged to test out the validity of the balanced thought through a behaviour experiment (see Chapter 10).

## Cognitive processes in MUS

We have discussed attentional focus and thinking errors earlier in the book, as they are fundamental to a formulation driven approach in CBT. The only time that these may not be considered is within a pure behavioural approach, where worry and rumination, for example, are viewed as behaviours. Traditional CBT would attend to content and processes in relation to cognitions associated with mental distress experienced by the patient. Even if it is at the level of acknowledgement of the presence of excessive worry and rumination, taking focus of attention to past experiences or uncertainty about the future, or attention focused on physical symptoms, therefore amplifying pain and associated emotional responses.

Table 12.1 presents common cognitive processes and how they may be affected in an MUS presentation.

### Working with cognitive processes

We have included examples of exercises designed to work with attentional focus in earlier chapters. In particular, in the chapter on working with depression and LTC (Chapter 5), we outlined mindfulness and ACT inspired techniques to bring

Table 12.1 Cognitive processes

| Cognitive process | Sub-categories | Description | Example in MUS |
|---|---|---|---|
| Attentional focus | Threat focus | When experiencing anxiety the mind goes onto threat-alert and the limbic system is activated. Once this occurs, the mind will actively search for the source of the threat. In the absence of a 'physical' threat – such as a violent intruder holding a gun to your head, or slipping off the top of a mountain – then the mind will draw conclusions as to what the threat is. | In response to a physical sensation associated with anxiety such as butterflies in the stomach, the person will do a full body scan looking for an explanation of the threat response in terms of their physical symptoms they associate with the MUS. For example, someone with FM may focus on their joints and muscles, which then exacerbates the sensations, which they interpret as threatening. |
| | Worry | Worry is a normal process, but when engaged in excessively it will cause symptoms of anxiety that will exacerbate any physical symptoms already experienced, such as pain or fatigue, through the extended freeze response that excessive worry produces. Muscular tension is a major symptom. | A stream of what ifs. . . ? Worst case scenarios are activated and this leads to some of the thinking errors listed as follows – in particular catastrophising and all or nothing thinking. Typical example would be when inactive due to pain or other symptoms, concluding they will never get better. |
| | Rumination | Although rumination is a normal thinking process, it is more frequent and enduring when there is either anxiety and/or depression symptoms as described earlier. Inactivity encourages excessive rumination, which is experienced as a continual loop of negative thoughts which tend to be focused on past events or current events that are perceived as 'problems' | A common ruminative theme in MUS is productivity (or lack of perceived productivity). Often the person will focus on what they used to be able to do and compare that with their present state. A 'before and after' dichotomy is set up, which leads to negative conclusions such as the activation of negative core beliefs such as 'I am a failure'. |

(Continued)

Table 12.1 (Continued)

| Cognitive process | Sub-categories | Description | Example in MUS |
|---|---|---|---|
| | Imagery | When on threat-alert it is common to experience the content of the threat in the form of an image. Worst case scenarios are played out over and over again, or traumatic memories are recalled as images which can make them feel as if they are reliving the events, or actively predicting what is going to happen to them. | Person experiences sensations of pain in their limbs and have images of being very active in the past, or images of themselves in a wheelchair in the future or both. |
| Thinking biases | All or nothing | What Beck describes as dichotomous thinking – or black and white thinking. The person will view information as being at one extreme or other, without being able to see 'shades of grey'. This thinking style is very rigid and leads to behaviours within the rules that are described in more detail as follows. | Struggling to complete a piece of coursework due to fatigue, the person will only be able to consider the possibility of doing the work to their usual high standard or failing. They will not be able to think of the possibility of scoring between a pass and a very high mark. |
| | Mental filter | According to Beck's original theory, and subsequent research in cognitive science, there is a negative thinking bias associated with depression. Even in anxiety disorders, the threat focus often ends up in a hopeless train of thought that triggers a more negative thinking style | Noticing a symptom after light work, initially makes the person worry 'what if I am never able to work at a higher level ever again?' This can lead to a sense of hopelessness and associated negative thoughts such as 'what's the point in trying?' or 'nothing will ever change' |
| | Over-generalisation | This cognitive bias has also been shown to be present in depression. In particular, with regard to memory. If one thing goes 'wrong' then this will be generalised to 'everything always goes wrong'. | A person with CFS had a difficult day last week when they couldn't complete a report at work. They now generalise that they never complete reports on time and may or may not attribute this to their condition. |

| Catastrophising | Catastrophic thinking is when you imagine the worst-case scenario or overestimate the level of threat of a particular thought or situation. This is common in all anxiety disorders. | Before going out for a meal with friends, someone with IBS may think about having an attack in the restaurant, ruining their meal and whole evening. Catastrophic thinking often leads to avoidance or excessive safety behaviours to try and prevent the feared event happening. |
|---|---|---|
| Personalisation | This is when negative events are attributed to something about you as a person. People who experience this thinking bias will often be hypervigilant to non-verbal expressions from other people – seeing them as evidence that the person is not happy with them, which leads to negative conclusions such as 'they don't like me' | A work colleague enters the room looking flustered and sighing loudly. You automatically assume it is someone you have done to upset them. This conclusion will be strengthened if you are suffering with difficult symptoms at that time, leading to a possible belief 'they are mad with me because I haven't worked hard enough today'. |

attention back to the present moment and focus on activities that are aligned with the person's values. We recommend that you refer back to that chapter for ideas for working with attentional focus.

With regard to thinking biases, these can be included within the psycho-education from the start of therapy. As with any cognitive therapy approach, the thinking biases will be introduced when working with NATs. Initially the person will be asked to identify the ones they recognise, then monitor them during any thought diary work. This is no different for when working with people with MUS. Just going through the common thinking styles in MUS may help to normalise this for them.

## Common rules in MUS

A key issue when working with cognitions is the relationship between beliefs, rules and negative thoughts. In the Beck approach, it is accepted that beliefs and rules are fundamental, and that negative thoughts arise from them, but the negative thoughts also have a role in reinforcing and maintaining them, as of course do the associated behaviours. (Sometimes the rules may 'stand-alone', without there being a clear dysfunctional core belief: a person may just believe that they should do things perfectly as this was strongly emphasised to them as a child, and they do not believe it has major consequence for them, or says anything about them as a person if they do not do things perfectly.) Usually, however, the rule has a clear relationship with a belief, often a defensive relationship, in that whilst the rule is being followed then the core belief with its associated emotion is not in the person's immediate awareness.

Following are the common rules for living we see presented in people with MUS.

### All or nothing

We have already stated that the all or nothing rule is the most common in people presenting with MUS, which accounts for the boom and bust behavioural pattern described in earlier chapters. We associate all or nothing rules with perfectionism, having unrelenting standards that are impossible to maintain. However, all or nothing rules can also be formulated in terms of completing tasks, regardless of standard. In these rules, it will be the lack of perceived productivity or completion of the excessive 'to do' list which results in the all or nothing pattern. For example, setting out to finish everything before lunch so that they can 'relax' the rest of the day creates a false sense of having to complete tasks before they can rest.

All or nothing rules can also be related to a sense of self-reliance, so doing everything yourself instead of asking for help or delegating gives a perceived sense of remaining in control. This inevitably results in the person with MUS doing more than they need to do at any time, which leads to not only physical exhaustion and a worsening of symptoms, but negative emotions such as resentment to others

*Table 12.2* Rules

| All or nothing rule | Function of the rule | Core belief activated if rule breaks | Example |
|---|---|---|---|
| If I can't do it perfectly, then there is no point in doing it | Gives a sense of maintaining high standards | I am a failure<br>I am not good enough<br>I am useless | Have a task to complete for work, but doesn't think there is enough time to complete it to their standard so they avoid it altogether and make an excuse. |
| If I can't complete the task, then there is no point in starting it | Completing tasks is viewed as the essence of productivity | I am a failure<br>I am not good enough<br>I am useless | The house is messy and needs cleaning but they are feeling too tired and in pain to do whole house so don't do anything. |
| If I push myself hard enough, then I can achieve anything | Gives a sense of maintaining self-reliance and control | I am weak<br>I am vulnerable<br>I am not good enough | Feeling tired and stressed but carries on working through the 'to do' list. |
| If I do everything now, then I can relax later | Working hard now to earn a reward later | I am weak<br>I am vulnerable | Looks around and can see more things that need doing, so carries on working before taking a rest |

or frustration with themselves for not being physically and emotionally able to complete all the tasks they set out to achieve. If it has a control function, then not completing tasks will feel threatening to the person – 'if I don't finish it now, then I will have to do it later but I am too exhausted already'. This then leads to avoidance and the associated rumination and worry.

## How to make all or nothing rules more flexible

These rules are incredibly rigid and commanding, and are probably one of the most difficult to change. This is because so much is at stake if we consider the function of the rule – to maintain high standards even when suffering, being productive, self-reliant and in control. These are all extremely important to a person whose ability to function is compromised, and who fear failure and view lack of productivity as a sign of weakness or uselessness. So even suggesting that these rules are not helpful and need changing is going to be very threatening.

The way we work with any rule is to not change it completely but to make it more flexible. With these rules we want to encourage 'all or nothing' to be adapted to 'little and often'. Not only is this a less taxing manner of approaching tasks, it still serves to protect the function of the current rule – that is, productivity, control and high standards – but it is the manner in which they perform the tasks which will change. So you can still clean the whole house, but in manageable sized time frames across more sessions. For example, instead of two hours in one go, try 30 minutes a day four times a week.

### Control rules

We have already established that some all or nothing rules have a control function, but another common rule is 'if I lose control, then something bad will happen'. This is relevant in terms of symptoms, as there is the fear that if they don't feel in control of them, then their condition will get worse. This leads to avoidance or being overcautious with activities, or the use of excessive safety behaviours to manage symptoms. Control is also associated with intolerance to uncertainty, which is clearly a common issue with MUS by their very nature.

### Subjugation rules

It is also common for people with MUS to put others before themselves, as we saw in the lived experience chapter written by Helen Moya. Being a 'doer' is part of the beliefs developed from childhood for various reasons. Being productive or having unrelenting standards can be driven by a need for approval. When they are unable to be productive, then there is a threat that others may reject them due to the belief that they are only accepted or approved of because they are so efficient.

*Table 12.3* Control rules

| Control rule | Function | Core beliefs activated if rule breaks | Example |
| --- | --- | --- | --- |
| If I lose control, then something bad will happen | Maintains a sense of self-management, and acceptance by others | I am weak<br>I am vulnerable | Asking for help risks judgement by others and possible rejection. |
| If I am not certain about everything, then things will get worse | Perceived sense of control by seeking information and reassurance from others (family and healthcare professionals) | I am weak<br>I am vulnerable | Asking lots of questions, researching on the internet, to make sure you know as much as possible about your symptoms. |

*Table 12.4* Subjugation rules

| Subjugation rule | Function | Core beliefs activated if rule breaks | Example |
|---|---|---|---|
| If I don't put others first, then I will be rejected | Maintains a sense of productivity and positive self-esteem by doing things for others, leading to perceived acceptance | I am not good enough Others are judgmental and critical | Pushing self to do things for all the family even when exhausted, to prevent criticism. |

## When to work with rules and beliefs

The conventional wisdom when treating straightforward disorders is to work initially with thoughts, and then to spend some sessions, if necessary, working with rules and beliefs with a relapse prevention rationale. There is a certain lack of sense here, because if these deeper cognitive processes need more sessions the work should not be allocated just a few sessions at the end of therapy. In actual clinical situations with MUS patients, it is the authors' experience that it is useful to work at this level quite early (the evidence base, however, does not provide much evidence as to whether it is helpful to work with rules/beliefs in MUS). There may be a case for working at this level and bypassing the negative thought level; this needs to be judged on an individual basis.

The first stage is to get the wording right, to ensure that the rule that you have agreed upon and written down is one that 'rings true' to the patient. (There are photocopy-able worksheets in Greenberger & Padesky, 2015.) Some clinicians use different forms for rules and for beliefs, but one type of form can cover both.

### 'Changing the rules' procedure and clinical example

Write the rule at the top of the sheet. Explore with the person that whether they agree that the rule is to some degree unhelpful or unreasonable, and contributes to symptoms. If the person is uncertain about this then discuss their strong allegiance to the rule suggesting ways in which it does not always serve them. Explain the rationale for doing this work, by saying, for example; 'Thinking back to the formulation that we did, you'll remember that we identified rules that were contributing to the problem. What I'd like to do now is to do some work on these, trying to help you make them more flexible and useful to you. It is important to say that we are not attacking your personality! We all have rules, most of which are helpful; it is important, however, to recognise how certain unhelpful rules contribute to the problems that you are having. It may be that the rules developed when you were younger to help you deal with a situation but they are less relevant now. What do you think of doing this?'

Start working through the questions on the form, asking the patient to read and respond to the questions. This has to be a slow and sensitive process, remembering that patients have adhered to these rules for a long time.

1) What is the old rule or belief?

2) P; 'I must always do things perfectly'

2) Where did the rule or belief come from and how has it been reinforced over the years?

P; 'My dad was a very successful businessman and had extremely high expectations of us, in all areas of our life. He was also quite critical, particularly of me, in comparison to my sisters who were prettier and cleverer. I took his criticisms to heart and it knocked my self-esteem. I felt the only way to get more love and praise from my dad was to be the best in absolutely everything and I guess I'm still like that'

It can be quite difficult and emotional for the patient to explore the basis of their assumption. However, it is important to have a full discussion of key factors. These may be parental attitudes, cultural and religious values, school experiences or relationships: sometimes the patient needs some encouragement in talking about these things. It can also help to explore the way that the rules have been reinforced, which can be a subtler issue. For example, the way that the successful implementation of the rule leads to a reward, the way that the rule stops the person acting in another way which stops them learning that the other way may be better.

3) What effect has the rule or belief had on your life?

P; 'I think when I was younger, I used to work extremely hard at school. It helped me get good A levels. When I got a job, it led me to always want to be the best, to get promotion and so on. More negatively it makes me set fantastic, unrealistic standards for myself, I'm exhausted I have a lot of pain. Having to be top saleswoman, never making mistakes, it's very tiring!' Even if I achieve these things, I'm not happy. The main advantage is that in some ways it helps me be successful at work; I've reached quite a senior position. That gives me a good income'

The therapist should acknowledge the benefits of the rule then explore the historic and current disadvantages of thinking like this. The clinician should acknowledge that the rule may have advantages, but could ask whether the advantages would occur if the person believed a modified version of the rule, for example, instead of believing that she must always do things perfectly, to have believed that she should aim to do her best, but accept that sometimes it will be impossible to achieve. The clinician should always ask what the patient's concerns are about giving up the rule.

4) How do I know the rule or belief is active?

P; 'I feel particularly tired. I also feel stressed if I'm aiming for something like a sales target and not reaching it. I can get a bit irritable with my boyfriend if he's getting in the way of what I want to do.' It is important to draw out as many factors as possible and relate them specifically to the rule.

5) What is the evidence that the rule or belief is not 100% true?

P; 'I'm not sure, possibly because it's impossible to do things perfectly. Or there's no such thing as perfection. In real life you've got to prioritise things.'

Here it is important to discuss as many arguments as possible that show that the rule is unrealistic. Typical questions would be;

- In what way is this rule unrealistic?
- Is there a law that says you must accept this?
- What would the world be like if everyone thought like this?

7) Why is the rule or belief unhelpful to me?

P; 'I feel incredibly stressed, anxious, I have lots of physical symptoms, pain and fatigue. I don't take enough time to rest. Possibly family life suffers a bit because I'm always late at work.'

Again, the therapist can ask a range of questions to elicit unhelpful side effects. For example:

'What adverse effect does the rule have on your mood, your physical symptoms, your thinking, your behaviour, your relationships, your work etc., (at the moment and in the past)?', 'How would you advise your best friend if they always followed this rule?'

The patient should be given a homework task of collecting evidence daily that runs contrary to the old belief or rule

8) What is the new rule or belief? (At this stage it is important to discuss with the patient what the new rule should be. It should reflect flexibility, therefore should express a 'preference' rather than a 'must;' it should lead to outcomes that are beneficial to the patient; it should be a statement that the person is happy to try to work on accepting; it should not be a statement that is too long and convoluted; it should reflect that following the rule is not likely to lead to disastrous outcomes).

P; 'I'll aim to do my best if it is an important issue. I will have to prioritise, issues and may not be able to give 100% effort, all the time'

9) Provide further evidence that the new rule or belief is more realistic and helpful?

P 'Since I've been trying to follow it, I haven't been staying so late. I've been getting slightly behind with my work but it's manageable. I was spending a lot of time before checking that I've not made mistakes, and it hasn't led to more mistakes.'

10) Devise behavioural changes/experiments that test or support the new rule or belief?

This is fundamentally important and is a process of moving the patient from a lightly held 'intellectual' acceptance of the rule, to a firmly held 'emotional' acceptance of the rule.

The key factor here will be devising behavioural changes or experiments, in which the person acts in accordance with the new rule. For example:

A    I will finish work at 6 pm on at least four days out of five.
B    When I am doing a final draft of my essay, I will take no longer than three hours.
C    When I am studying my university course I will not procrastinate. I will start working within five minutes of sitting at the desk.
D    Next month I will aim to be the second top salesperson, and not first as I usually do.

The helpfulness and acceptability of the behaviours and the effect on the new rule, would be reviewed every session.

## Core beliefs in MUS

Core beliefs according to Beck (1976) are the fundamental and rigidly held beliefs that are formed in response to early experiences. His early work on cognitive therapy for depression described what he called the cognitive triad, which are beliefs about self, others and the future. Later proponents of cognitive therapy such as Padesky, include beliefs about the world, which are very useful when trying to understand the onset and development of the person's presenting problems in CBT.

Like many conditions, there are a variety of possible core beliefs that people with MUS may hold. This will depend on a number of factors in relation to their early experiences. There is often an assumption that it is only negative core beliefs that contribute to the experience of having MUS. Examples include: I am weak, I am vulnerable, I am not good enough. However, it can be the case that a person has grown up with very positive beliefs which then become shattered when they experience symptoms that prevent them from maintaining their adaptive beliefs about self. For example, in the case of being a high achiever throughout school and career, with the core belief 'I am competent', on experiencing a debilitating condition which results in reduced functioning this belief may shatter.

We need to make a judgement as to whether the core beliefs are impacting on the medical unexplained symptoms in some way. If this is the case, we are likely to work on this, if we have the time to do so, there is a collaborative formulation in place that identifies this as a salient issue, and there is a good therapeutic relationship. The standard way of doing this is thought continuum work, building up healthy schemas, positive date log, and experiential techniques such as imagery (Padesky, 2020).

### Continuum log

The rationale of the continuum log would be to break down black and white thinking. If we take a belief that is core to the person that they have had since adolescence, namely, 'doctors get it wrong, and that puts me in danger', this belief arose from a serious misdiagnosis when the person was a teenager.

*T:*   Would you be willing to work on this belief?
*P:*   I will, but it seems quite scary to give up.
*T:*   I understand this, because of what's happened to you, but we agreed it's causing you problems now. I don't want to put you in any danger I just want to help you think clearly about things. We can use a technique called continuum. Let's put your belief at one end of the continuum. What's the more balance believe that we could put out the other end?
*P:*   They can sometimes get it right
*T:*   what I want to do now is to break this down into more specific instances of this.

The therapist then breaks down the issue of doctors getting it right or not right into more specific examples such as getting it right about diagnosis, getting it right treatment wise, getting medication right, getting it right interpersonally. It may be then helpful to get the person to read it to be is on a continuum, perhaps with the questions such as how often do you think to get a diagnosis rate, how often do you think to get medication right. Patient may accept this or say that their mistakes are potentially serious or fatal. This may lead to further continuum or discussion around how many fatal mistakes occur in each medical interaction. The next stage could be look at this historically, by looking at specific examples of interactions that did not have a mistake in them. Or the patient could do a survey around the level of mistakes and GP interactions that people have experienced. Or they could make a record of every time they have been to the GP and whether a mistake was made.

### Positive data log

The rationale here is to collate evidence that undermines the old belief and/or supports the new belief. In terms of the aforementioned example, the patient could keep a daily record of interactions with health professionals and whether serious mistakes were made. The positive data log can also be used to make any general negative core beliefs more flexible. For example, if the person has a rigid core belief 'I am not good enough', which is driving their rule to push themselves hard, then completing a positive data log looking for evidence against this belief can be encouraged. Be clear what sounds as data. The following list are some examples:

• Compliments
• If someone smiles at you for no particular reason
• If someone asks how you are
• When you notice that you have done something you are proud of
• Noticing when you have made an effort even if you didn't complete all the task
• Doing nice things without having to 'earn them' by working hard

Positive data logs can be completed in different media. Keeping a note book and jotting down observations may not always be practical, so other suggestions include: using notes app on phone, taking photos of the data to look back on and reflect, or drawing items. The reflecting back over all the logged data is an important aspect of the procedure as this provides an opportunity to demonstrate how much information normally gets filtered out during each day. By noticing it daily, a pathway to this information is made more flexible, as opposed to automatically going to the negative information that reinforces the negative core belief.

### Experiential techniques

Experiential techniques such as imagery or empty chair (Pugh, 2018) can help with emotional expression, dealing with past traumatic events, strengthening up cognitive work. The patient here could do an empty chair exercise on one chair playing the belief that 'doctors get it wrong and that puts me in danger' then swap into the opposite chair playing the new belief, always, of course, finishing on the new belief. An alternative to this would be going back to the incident of the misdiagnosis, and doing an interaction between the mistaken GP and the patient, with a view to emotional processing, change of perspective, clarifying the accuracy of the memory, expressing thoughts and feelings, etc.

### Building up healthy core beliefs

The final stage is to agree a new belief, for example 'Doctors usually get it right, but occasionally can make mistakes, with various consequences, which I can safeguard against by questioning them'. This needs to be road-tested by the use of flashcards, continuation of already practice techniques and specifically collecting information through a positive data log. The patient must address the unhelpful behaviours that arise from the belief, in order to strengthen it: in this example it may include constantly seeking for second opinions, avoiding the GP, or going excessively, selectively attending to only certain things that the GP says etc. The patient changes these behaviours to strengthen the new core belief. A way to measure change is to rate how much they believe the new belief on a scale of 0–100% at each therapy appointment. Because this is the core belief this will take persistence and patience on the part of the therapist and the patient, some beliefs being more amenable to change than others.

## Chapter summary

Medically unexplained symptoms can be maintained by negative thoughts: negative processes such as worry, rumination and thinking errors; also rules for a living and core beliefs.

These probably have their effect through impact on mood and emotion, and through unhelpful behavioural patterns. Standard CBT approaches can be used including: challenging negative thoughts, making worries and rumination more concrete, changing the rules through utilising the rule sheet and through behavioural experiments. With core beliefs, continuum work, imagery and flashcards can be used over an extended period of therapy. The formulation should guide at what level you work with cognition, particularly as the evidence base as to the specific problematic conditions that patients have is weak.

## Chapter 13

# Aiding patients with emotional expression and regulation

There is a comprehensive literature on the impact of emotional factors on MUS. These would include the impact of *alexithymia*, the role of *negative affectivity* and *anxiety/depression* presenting as medically unexplained symptoms.

## Alexithymia

The word derives from the Greek, and means not having a language of emotion. The most influential way of understanding this, which has broadly stood the test of time (Preece, Becerra, Allan, Robinson & Dandy, 2017), is the work of Taylor, Ryan and Bagby (1985) who identified the key elements of: difficulty identifying emotions, difficulty describing feelings and externally orientated thinking, and many studies have used his Toronto scale to measure these constructs. Research has provided indications of alexithymia causing problems across all emotion response systems, subjective, physiological and behavioural, and across all stages of emotion processing, including initial perception, response and regulation (Luminet, Rimé, Bagby & Taylor, 2004; Pollatos & Gramann, 2011). It is also now generally accepted that alexithymia is associated with psychosomatic disorder, independent of depression and anxiety, a large population study of over 5,000 patients showing this (Mattila et al., 2008), and this is supported in other studies. It has also been found that alexithymia patients have higher resting cardiovascular activity, and their immune systems are weaker. Patients with alexithymia are more likely to report symptoms than controls (one suggestion is that they may not be more ill, just more likely to seek help). Alexithymia is most helpfully seen as a both a trait and a state phenomenon (Lumley, Neely & Burger, 2007).

Tominaga, Choi, Nagoshi, Wada and Fukui (2014) evaluated the coping strategies of somatoform disorder patients with alexithymia, and they found problems with their coping strategies. Tominaga et al. (2014) found that the Difficulty Identifying Feeling (DIF) subscale of the Toronto Alexithymia Inventory was associated with the emotional escape – avoidance coping strategy which is consistent with previous research on somatoform disorder. Patients with a high DIF score are unable to discern emotions from somatic sensations. Also, the study found patients with high difficulty describing feelings (DDF) scores may have trouble

DOI: 10.4324/9780367824433-17

with social interactions, and lack interpersonal understanding, which may lead to lower social functioning; in turn, the patient may be less likely to seek social support and less likely to communicate their problems to others.

Again, in this study, the externally oriented thinking (EOT) score was strongly related to a non-confrontive coping strategy. EOT is characterised by action-oriented thinking that focuses on the factual aspects of external reality rather than on the psychological experience. Individuals with high EOT scores are less likely to cope with the stress of intractable problems (i.e., they are less likely to seek the elimination of the source with confidence). The more infrequent use of a confrontative/problem-solving strategy may be partly due to difficulty in discerning the source of the stress and confidently working toward a solution. Thus, for patients with high EOT scores, useful intervention approaches may include techniques that promote the understanding that physical symptoms can be related to the stressful situation and techniques that aid in identifying the cause of the problem (Tominaga et al., 2014).

Another useful suggestion is that the broad construct of alexithymia contains at least two subtypes (Larsen, Brand, Bermond & Hijman, 2003); Type 1 alexithymia refers to the classic alexithymic person who has little experience or display of emotion, minimal emotional awareness and verbalisation, and a pronounced external orientation. Such people are emotionally neutral or bland; place little value on psychological processes; and relate to others in a rigid, machine-like fashion. In contrast, the so-called Type 2 alexithymic person experiences and expresses heightened levels of negative emotion but has difficulty identifying and labelling his or her own feelings and is confused, overwhelmed, feels numb, or acts out when aroused (Lumley et al., 2007). The authors of this book feel that this separation is clinically valid.

It has also been suggested that alexithymia can also be considered as a type of emotional avoidance where the person learns to consistently avoid distressing emotional experience and the relief he gets reinforces the avoidant strategies (Panayiotou et al., 2015)

The possible origins of emotional avoidance or alexithymia could be early experiences (for example being brought up in a family in which talking about feelings is not normal or acceptable); individual biological variation; cultural factors; and history of trauma, where the person has learned to numb their feelings (Butler & Surawy, 2004). Cognitions here are potentially in three areas:

- *The meaning of having feelings*, that they are being weak, they will lose control or be overwhelmed, that the feelings will continue or get worse and result in some catastrophic state such as severe depression.
- *The meaning of expressing feelings*, the fear of being evaluated as weak, silly, childish a burden, or incomprehensible
- *Confusion about feelings*, that they cannot understand them, differentiate one from the other, or differentiate them from physical sensations (Butler & Surawy, 2004).

How do you detect and measure alexithymia, and decide whether to address it?

In detecting this, we would look out for patients, who are more likely to be male, and who tend to not express their emotions strongly, they may not have a language of emotion, and they may be unduly logical. If you ask about their feelings, they may discuss physical symptoms. They may identify with underlying rules such as, 'if you show emotion . . . you are weak . . . you will lose control . . . you will be punished.' The main specific features of alexithymia to look out are: (1) difficulty identifying feelings, and distinguishing them from bodily sensations, (2) difficulty describing feelings to others and (3) externally oriented thinking (thinking that is focused on the details and facts of the situation rather than the psychological aspects). Alexithymic patients tend not to use complex or nuanced emotional language but are more likely to express themselves in bodily symptoms or provide excessive details of their health, daily events, or actions. Such communication should not be viewed as a secondary gain strategy or avoidance of effort or commitment. One can question as to whether these patients need specific work on emotional regulation and expression: this will depend on the clinician's formulation, and whether the process of alexithymia directly impacts on the psychosomatic symptoms. A recently large trial (Kleinstäuber et al., 2019) did not show any differences between standard and emotionally enhanced CBT, though it could be argued that the two interventions were not vastly different. This study may be evidence that standard CBT is enough in MUS, to at least bring about some change. One study showed that active treatment of alexithymia can reduce it and had an impact on cardiovascular disease (Beresnevaite, 2000), but treatment research and strategy is undeveloped.

### How do you treat alexithymia?

All these techniques need to be applied using the standard CBT principles of collaboration and guided discovery: Lumley, Neely and Burger (2007) hypothesise that coping skills training, including techniques such as relaxation, pleasant activity scheduling, distraction, activity-rest cycling and communication skills, might be particularly useful for people with alexithymia. Biofeedback may also be helpful not only because an external device helps patients reduce and manage arousal but also because it might teach patients the links between psychological states and physiological reactions.

Emotion work: the types of strategies that could be used, would be emotional awareness training, and emotional expression training. Let's look at these in turn: the first step of emotional awareness would be explaining the concept of emotions. The therapist could say: 'Emotions are biological processes associated with thoughts, bodily sensations and behaviours. We all have different degrees of awareness of these emotional states. If you have problems with medically unexplained symptoms this may be associated with how you handle these emotions. The problem could be poor awareness of emotion, or poor management of the thoughts feelings and behaviours associated with them. It may particularly be the case that this process contributes to your experience of the medically unexplained symptoms. The way this happens is not fully understood, but poor awareness (often called alexithymia) may cause emotional responses to be interpreted as physical symptoms or the signals that the emotions give you that something is bad or stressful may be ignored and the situation may continue to harm you. What do you think of this idea?' The therapist then goes on to explore the patient's views.

The next step would be to help the patient increase emotional awareness through tracking emotional responses, and keeping a diary of these. The therapist may have to initiate a discussion as to what emotions are (sadness, happiness, guilt) and what the patient's experience is of them. A further discussion could be around the history of having a particular experience of an illness, contrasted with having any emotional experience. The patient may have to be educated about typical words people use for emotion and they may have to understand the triggers that evoke an emotional experience. Another strategy could be a reliving of an *emotional incident* in a deep way: the patient is asked firstly to remember a happy (then a difficult experience): 'could you go over that happy/difficult incident again (in the present tense, first person, using your five senses). Can you focus on the emotion you are feeling during it, if it feels like a physical sensation would you able to say that may be an emotion (such as happiness, joy, excitement, sadness, anxiety, guilt, shame, anger)?'

The therapist could also make the therapy more emotionally focused in the session. This would mean that the therapist would draw attention to any sign of emotion in the session and encourage the patient to notice it, sit with it, describe it and process it. Experiences that could trigger off this strategy would be: any signs of anxiety or sadness that the patient displays; any description of a stressful or emotional incident, and a focus on a physical symptom. Potential responses from the therapist could be 'tell me more about that; how does it feel emotionally; is that physical sensation like any emotion; how does that feel in your body; how is it when I am asking you to focus on this?' A mindfulness approach, like the body scan, where the individual sits and slowly notices what bubbles up from his body or feelings can build tolerance and awareness (Segal & Teasdale, 2018). Researchers such as Lieberman, Inagaki, Tabibnia and Crockett (2011), Craske, Hermans and Vervliet (2018) have found that affect labelling, may be helpful for emotional processing. In doing this, we would agree some homework with the patient that when they met a situation that they or others would describe as difficult (or positive), then the patient should, out loud, label and describe the emotion that they have, for example 'I'm going for our job interview, I've got a headache, this could be anxiety, anxiety is like a pain in the head, I've had anxiety like this before our job interviews.'

Behaviours and avoidance: If a consequence of alexithymia is that the person tends to ignore or avoid stressors (by not realising the emotional effects they are having on them), the therapist could try, 'how do you respond to stress . . . can you acknowledge it . . . do you just like to get on with things . . . do you avoid issues?' It may be that the idea from Dugas and Robichaud's approach to GAD is useful here, the idea of negative problem orientation, that patients may not particularly be bad at dealing with problems when they do face them but may tend to not address or recognise problems.

The person may have style of behaviourally avoiding stressful situations, thereby not learning to deal with them, or they may be, to use the ACT terminology, be experientially avoidant (Bilotta, Giacomantonio, Leone, Mancini & Coriale, 2016), we can consider as to whether alexithymia is a trait that occurs mostly out of awareness or something the person is using more strategically. The therapist could ask what the person is avoiding and set up experiments in facing it testing their fears. Given that these patients do not seek social support, then examining this and helping patients do it is helpful.

Cognitive: this can be approached at the level of content and process. A potential problem in using the negative thought diary, is that the use of this is triggered by noticing an emotion, so this would have to be done after extensive education about emotional awareness. It is more likely that we will work at the level of core beliefs and rules for living, some of which are noted earlier and can be elicited by assessment and questionnaire. 'Rules for living' are best tackled by using the relevant form (see Chapter 9), helping the patient work through: where the rule came from, how it is affecting them, how it does not match the way the world works, culminating in the development of a new flexible rule, and behavioural experiments to test this out: 'If I don't keep my emotions under control, it is humiliating, or the feeling won't stop', 'I need to keep my emotions hidden, or I am in danger'. Core beliefs such as, 'emotions are shameful', or 'emotions are dangerous' can be approached in the standard way, which is putting emotions on a continuum, looking historically at exceptions to these beliefs, collecting evidence on a day-to-day basis that the beliefs are not true or helpful. Empty chair or imagery techniques could be used here. For example, the patient could sit on a chair, and be the chair who believes 'Emotions are dangerous', describes this position, then moves onto the other chair, and argues for 'emotions are safe and natural, and can help me live a happy life' defending each point of view but finishing on the most helpful one. Early experiences that have led to the development of the belief 'emotions are dangerous', could be worked on with standard imagery techniques. For example, the patient in imagination, revisit these experiences, and challenges incidents that led to the development of the belief (Pugh, 2018)

In terms of communication, alexithymic individuals show problems in emotional language production and comprehension, in particular, display a limited ability to talk about interpersonal relationships, describe others' emotional experiences, and understand the emotions of others (Samur et al., 2013). Possible strategies could be to get patients to do these things, for example talk about close relationships in a personal and expressive way, either in session or doing an account as homework, doing an expressive writing task, in which something is written about using emotional and personal language, the patient could be asked to read a poem or novel or watch a film that would have an emotional content and describe his reaction to it. The Toronto questionnaire has a section on externally oriented thinking. If this is present the person could be asked to describe a situation in a personal way using the first person, present tense, describing how they react to it through their five senses and their emotions, and limiting factual aspects of the situation

## Attentional processes

If the patient is naturally moving their attention away from emotion then they may be trained to better recognise emotional expressions in faces (see Cook, Brewer, Shah & Bird, 2013) for a relevant task) and to have better recollection of emotional memories (see Luminet et al., 2004).

### Step-by-step approach to help with alexithymia

Identify alexithymia through assessment and questionnaire, (the best questionnaire is the Toronto alexithymia scale, it needs to be purchased)

Possible questions would be: 'How are you at expressing your feelings?', 'What feelings do you tend to have?', 'what goes through your mind when you think about showing your feelings?', 'if you don't show your feelings, what do you tend to do to keep them under control?',

Example:

*T:* Is it OK to ask you some questions about your feelings?
*P:* Okay
*T:* How are you expressing your feelings?
*P:* Probably not particularly good. I tried to keep things under control
*T;* Tell me about that
*T:* I don't want to be a burden. When I've said I felt down in the past people seem to respond negatively. I've got a feeling that if I say 'I'm struggling', people won't be interested or they'll walk out on me. If I notice I feel sad I just push it of my mind and get on with things.

So here they may be a degree of alexithymia or emotional avoidance that could be problematic.

Next stage is to try and understand whether the alexithymia is related to the medically unexplained symptoms the person is presenting.

Example continued:

*T:* Do you think when you don't express your feelings it could be related to your current symptoms?
*P:* I'm not sure
*T:* Could it be the case that not being so aware stops you dealing with the problems at the time as often your emotions are telling you that there is something wrong?

*P:* Maybe

*T:* Can you think of an example when this was the case
(Discussion of example)

*T:* is it possible that you experience something that is part of emotion, as a physical symptom or condition?

*P:* I'm not sure

*T:* Could we explore this, thinking of examples?

*P:* I'll try.

Here we might look for examples when the person avoided his feelings or experienced them as a symptom. The pattern of avoidance and alexithymia may make this quite difficult to do.

Further strategies for alexithymia are *increased emotional awareness*, which could be approached as follows:

• Discuss whether a pattern of emotional awareness would help.
• Goals will be negotiated with the patient, but potentially could be: 'I will be more aware when I have an emotion such as happiness, sadness, anger. I will acknowledge it and consider what may be contributing to it. If I have a physical symptom that is not explained by medical disease, and has been investigated by my GP, I will consider whether this could be part of an emotion.' Specific strategies could be:

a   Education about different emotions, what may typically trigger them off, what might be typical physical sensations. The 'wheel of emotions' is a useful resource here, if perhaps complicated.
b   This leads naturally on to the patient keeping a diary, such as the following:

*Table 13.1* Emotion diary

| Emotion diary: What emotion do I feel or have observed? How would I rate it 0–100%? | What has triggered it? | What physical sensations come with the emotion? | What did I do in response to the emotion? |
| --- | --- | --- | --- |
| | | | |
| | | | |
| | | | |
| | | | |
| | | | |

c    Use a technique such as the 'Changing the rules form' to challenge unhelpful attitudes to emotion which could be 'If I show or express my emotions, it will get out of control . . . I'll be rejected . . . the feeling won't stop . . . it's selfish . . . It's unmanly.' The goal will be to develop a more flexible attitude to emotion and try this out behaviourally. How this is done will be influenced by what the person does or avoids doing in an attempt to be emotionally avoidant: push thoughts out of mind, change subjects of conversation, dampen feelings down by experiences close to dissociation, avoid expressing emotions, for example by never saying 'I care for you . . . you're a great friend . . . I love you. . . .' (Some patients will only avoid uncomfortable emotions and others will avoid happy emotions.). If patients are avoiding situations that trigger feeling then they could experiment with facing them.

d    In the session the therapist could pay particular attention to emotionally laden moments. They could sensitively say, 'you seem affected by this. . . . I'm not sure if you were a little uncomfortable . . . I like the way you're being true to yourself; what emotion are you feeling. . . . I feel more connected to you when you are true to yourself. When you have that emotion how do you feel in your body? Are these sensations typical of the way you feel?'

e    The patient could be asked to pick a happy experience and describe it as if it was happening now, identifying their thoughts, feelings and physical sensations. This could be debriefed with the aim of encouraging emotional awareness and expression. The patient could then be asked to describe a sad or stressful experience.

f    Homework could then be negotiated in terms of taking this learning forward.

## Negative affect

Negative affect simply means that there is an elevated level of negative emotions like anxiety and depression, and the studies have shown that this is high in medically unexplained symptoms. Several interesting studies have suggested that negative affect is more important than alexithymia, in the expression of MUS. For example, Rief et al. (1996) showed that the association between alexithymia and the number of somatoform symptoms in 174 inpatients of a psychosomatic hospital disappeared when it was corrected for the possible impact of depression (i.e. negative affect). In line with this finding, Lane, Carroll, Ring, Beevers and Lip (2002) showed that patients with conversion disorder, functional somatic syndromes and medical controls did not differ in terms of 'Theory of Mind', emotional awareness or alexithymia after adjusting for positive and negative affect. One study found that alexithymia and neuroticism were stable personality states over six months, whereas negative affectivity was quite variable in this group (De Gucht, 2003).

As others have noted, it feels contradictory that it is postulated that MUS patients could potentially have elevated levels of anxiety and depression (negative affect) and also alexithymia, where emotion is not expressed. It is possible that some patients have both elevated levels of anxiety depression and an alexithymia style that leads to poor recognition, and emotional processing of these states. Or it may be that with the majority of patients the problem is high negative affectivity, and there is a smaller group of patients with alexithymia as a problem; this would be a clinical observation. Most of the patients we see come across as fairly stressed and anxious and about the symptoms, and we would see a smaller group of patients who are more controlled and distant in a typical alexithymic way. This may be a manifestation of the two types of alexithymia mentioned earlier (Larsen et al., 2003).

In summary, if patients have high affectivity then that is something we need to address, and all other chapters in this book have ideas how to do this, drawn from the CBT repertoire, and these would include building a therapeutic relationship, setting goals, doing a formulation, helping patients challenge negative automatic thoughts, change rules and beliefs, change unhelpful behaviours, engage in behavioural experiments, problem solve better, change the focus of attention, etc.

## Psychogenic non-epileptic seizures as a dysregulated emotion

Psychogenic non-epileptic seizures (PNES), are a condition in which sufferers have seizures (episodes of altered awareness), but have had epilepsy or other causes excluded by a neurologist, and the seizures have a significant impact in terms of distress, disability, loss of income and iatrogenic harm. Between 12% and 20% of adults presenting in epilepsy clinics have dissociative seizures (Goldstein et al., 2020). Three-quarters of patients with PNES are initially misdiagnosed and treated for epilepsy, which exposes patients to multiple iatrogenic harms and prevents them from accessing psychological treatment (which there is some evidence for the effectiveness, see Oto & Reuber, 2014). Seventy-five per cent of sufferers are women, a large proportion are socially deprived, and the main poor prognosis factor is duration of the condition, also receipt of benefits and general psychopathology (Goldstein et al., 2019).

The authors' experience is that patients will present with different degrees of loss of awareness, ranging from being spaced out, to losing consciousness (briefly). Patients may collapse to the ground, but if they have warnings of the seizure they can usually sit or lie down, so broken bones and serious injuries are possible but unusual. Incontinence is unusual but can happen. When patients awake, they are usually groggy for seconds to minutes (to hours). Patients usually keep a normal colour during the episode, and are not cyanosed. If a patient has an episode whilst the therapist is with them, she can speak to them and help ground them and sometimes stop the seizure. The cause of this condition is not fully understood; many patients have a history of sexual abuse, but not all. For CBT we would do a thorough assessment identifying predisposing, precipitating and maintenance factors. There is some evidence that dissociation is an important maintenance factor in generating the seizures (Grünewald, 2019), the response to traumatic memory or a stressful or physically painful experience in which the person blanks out to protect themselves from further distress; clinically this does make sense; however, there is a group who do not describe stressful triggering events, indeed no obvious triggers at all, and this is puzzling. It is not clear whether this lack of triggering event is related to alexithymia, shame around trauma and abuse, or some other obscure explanation. Our observations, having seen a lot of patients, is that the PNES can have quite an impact on their lives, especially if they are having many seizures throughout the day. Sometimes it is straightforward to identify trauma, stress, physical pain or other triggers, and there is a clear relationship to the seizure event.

The CBT approach is in two phases: the first phase is grounding and stabilisation, to reduce the seizures and the impact of them. The second phase is to deal with the triggering event. In terms of grounding, this works if the patient has a warning for the seizure, so they can be prepared with a grounding technique, and if there is no warning this makes therapy a lot harder. The grounding technique used would be negotiated with the patient; the rationale is based on reducing dissociation and bringing the patient back to the here and now: they will be asked to orientate himself to be present by saying something agreed like 'My name is James, it is Thursday afternoon I am sitting in the hospital, I am safe'. Sometimes a technique akin to the discrimination technique in the treatment of PTSD is helpful, where the person records the differences between the trauma event and what is happening in the real world at the moment. The person can physically ground himself to the chair he is sitting in, by feeling the fabric of the chair, his bottom on the seat, his back against the rear of the chair. The person can use a grounding object, and this would be something that relates to the person's present life and feels like a safe object; this could be a bangle or a stone; they could physically hold onto this when they felt the seizure coming on. They could also use a grounding smell that they associate with safety, such as rosewater, or perfume. In planning this, the therapist should go along with what the patient thinks will work best. An important consideration is that there will only be seconds to minutes for the patient to use a grounding technique, so they need to use it rapidly at the first sign of an impending seizure. It is hoped and expected that this technique will stop the seizure happening: experience is that this will happen in perhaps 50% of cases. Occasionally patients will say that if they stop the seizure it builds up, and will occur again later, and if this is the case the technique is best avoided. This technique is done in conjunction with establishing what the key triggers are, so the patient is ready to use it.

From a behavioural perspective we would encourage patients to take 'safe risks'; what we mean by that is to start going out into the world, and gradually doing normal activities. In planning this, we would try to ensure that they would not be harmed by things that could be genuinely dangerous to them, the obvious examples being having a bath, crossing the road in busy traffic and driving a car. There is a delicate balance in helping the person do things that help rehabilitate them, and they have been excessively avoiding, but ensuring that they are not in any actual danger, and this needs to be done collaboratively. (The older behavioural model viewed NES as purely being reinforced by family attention, and the relief from escaping activities, but we think this is too simplistic.)

The second part of the therapy is dealing with the triggering event. If it is a traumatic event, then normal CBT approaches such as exposure, relieving and EMDR can be used. Our experience is that traumas (in the context of non-epileptic seizures) respond well to this approach. Sometimes the trigger is physical pain, so we try to understand and reduce the impact of this. Sometimes it is stressful life events, and we use a range of CBT techniques such as problem-solving, setting goals and challenging negative thoughts.

### The interaction between MUS and anxiety/depression

The other emotional issue to think about is misunderstanding patients as having some type of psychosomatic disorder, when they really have a depression or anxiety disorder. The situation arises when the patient persistently presents symptoms such as tiredness, headache, chest pain, muscle pain etc. and although one may initially suspect a type of psychosomatic disorder, after questioning it is clear that the presenting problem is depression or a specific anxiety disorder, and this should become clear when a thorough assessment is done. The patient will describe their panic or low mood as a key problem and the physical symptoms will be directly related to this problem, in the sense that they will arise from, and be strongly associated with their depression and anxiety. Furthermore, they will score highly on specific measures of depression and anxiety disorders, and will have a fairly typical cognitive profile, for example in depression, themes of loss, lack of enjoyment in life, withdrawal and avoidance associated. In this case we would expect that a treatment of their anxiety or depressive disorder with psychological or pharmacological methods would eventually relieve the physiological symptoms.

## Chapter summary

Alexithymia, which means not having a word for emotion, is implicated in medically unexplained symptoms. Patients typically have problems identifying and describing emotion, and think in an external way. They may have beliefs and rules which drive this. Once this has been identified, techniques such as emotional labelling, expressive writing, tracking emotions, facing situations, sitting with emotions can be used within the session and as homework. Negative affect, which means high anxiety and/or depression, is also associated with medically unexplained symptoms, and can be treated with normal CBT techniques. Another thing to consider is that the symptoms may be medically unexplained, but in some cases are really a symptom of a primary anxiety or depression condition.

# Chapter 14

# Identifying and helping patients who are fearful of recovery

## Understanding fear of recovery/secondary gain

The issue of the best term to describe this phenomenon is delicate: secondary gain can be used, or *fear of recovery* (FOR); the latter is the one we prefer and will use from now on, as it is less pejorative, but we will occasionally refer to secondary gain as it is commonly used. (Most authorities would differentiate this secondary gain or fear of recovery from *malingering*, where there is a deliberate and conscious feigning of illness this can occur in a calculated way to achieve financial or other benefits. A further (uncommon) presentation is *factitious disorder* where the person feigns physical, or less commonly psychological illness, usually to meet a need of being cared for (Kinsella, 2001).)

Nevertheless, mainstream clinical opinion and the research literature agree that some patients with MUS are fearful of getting better. The original concept of secondary gain comes originally from Freud (Van Egmond, 2003): it originally meant that patients will have social or interpersonal benefits from having symptoms, and contrasts, in Freudian terms with primary gain, where there is an emotional gain from the illness presentation. From a learning theory perspective, the behaviour of having symptoms leads to reward in not having to go to work, or in obtaining benefits or compensation, or experiencing a distressing situation, the behaviour is thus negatively re-enforced, and so continues. In one interesting study, over 300 patients were treated on an inpatient psychosomatic service employing a learning model of chronic illness behaviour. This model stressed the role of social reinforcement and avoidance of occupational and social activities, in the maintenance of a medically unexplained syndrome. Preliminary studies showed that patients naturally reinforced others for care-giving responses but showed improved tolerance of experimental pain, and lower rates of medication use, when care-taking responses were minimised and self-control encouraged. Patients who return to an intact family show continuing decreases in somatic complaints and increases in achievement orientation, and treatment failures were characterised by lack of an intact family, and return to the medical care system (Wooley, Blackwell & Winget, 1978). This study is therefore some evidence about the negative effect of encouraging illness behaviours.

DOI: 10.4324/9780367824433-18

In another study, Craig et al. (1994), showed that in the 38 weeks prior to symptoms occurring, somatisers (MUS) were more likely to have an event that had the potential for secondary gain. In a further study, 60% of patients with psychogenic movement disorders had an activating event and a possible secondary gain element like a compensation claim (Factor, Podskalny & Molhno, 1995). Across diagnoses, with patients in therapy the prospects of gaining something external from the therapy lead to poorer outcomes (Van Egmond & Kummeling, 2002). Patients in the German psychosomatic rehabilitation centre, who are 'neurotic patients' who wish to retire early from work, over-reported their symptoms at a rate of 18.8%; moreover extended times of sick leave and higher expectations of disability pension are associated with elevated non-credible symptom endorsement, and this was viewed to be influenced by secondary gain. Patients who elevate their symptoms have poorer outcomes (Merten, Kaminski & Pfeiffer, 2019). A major review of the secondary gain concept (Fishbain, Rosomoff, Cutler & Rosomoff, 1995) summarised that the results of the reviewed studies support the potential importance of the 'secondary gain' concept to understanding illness behaviour, and underscore a need for future research in this area.

This delicate issue of fear of recovery/secondary gain, which may be conscious or out of awareness, will be discussed here in terms of contextual factors such as family dynamics, work experiences, interactions with benefit systems, fearfulness, re-enforcement etc.

### How can the therapist establish whether this is present?

- The symptoms do not seem as severe as the patient is stating, though there may be other reasons for this.
- There is a very attentive spouse or family.
- There is a history of dependent traits.
- Financial benefits are available that would make getting well very disadvantageous.
- The patient's history is inconsistent or hard to understand.
- If the patient improved, they would have to return to a difficult situation.

So, we can see that this patient faced with some secondary gain, and the possibility of recovering from their symptoms, has a number of thoughts, which may or may not be in full awareness, leading to anxiety, more focus on symptoms, further cognitions, emotions and negative and unhelpful behaviours. The common patterns that we have seen in clinical practice are as follows, and again in saying this we are not stating these apply to all patients and are not being judgemental of those where they are present:

- The patient does not want to go back to work because they dislike their job, or it was a major source of stress that made them ill in the first place
- The person is on sickness or disability benefits which they will lose if their symptoms clear up

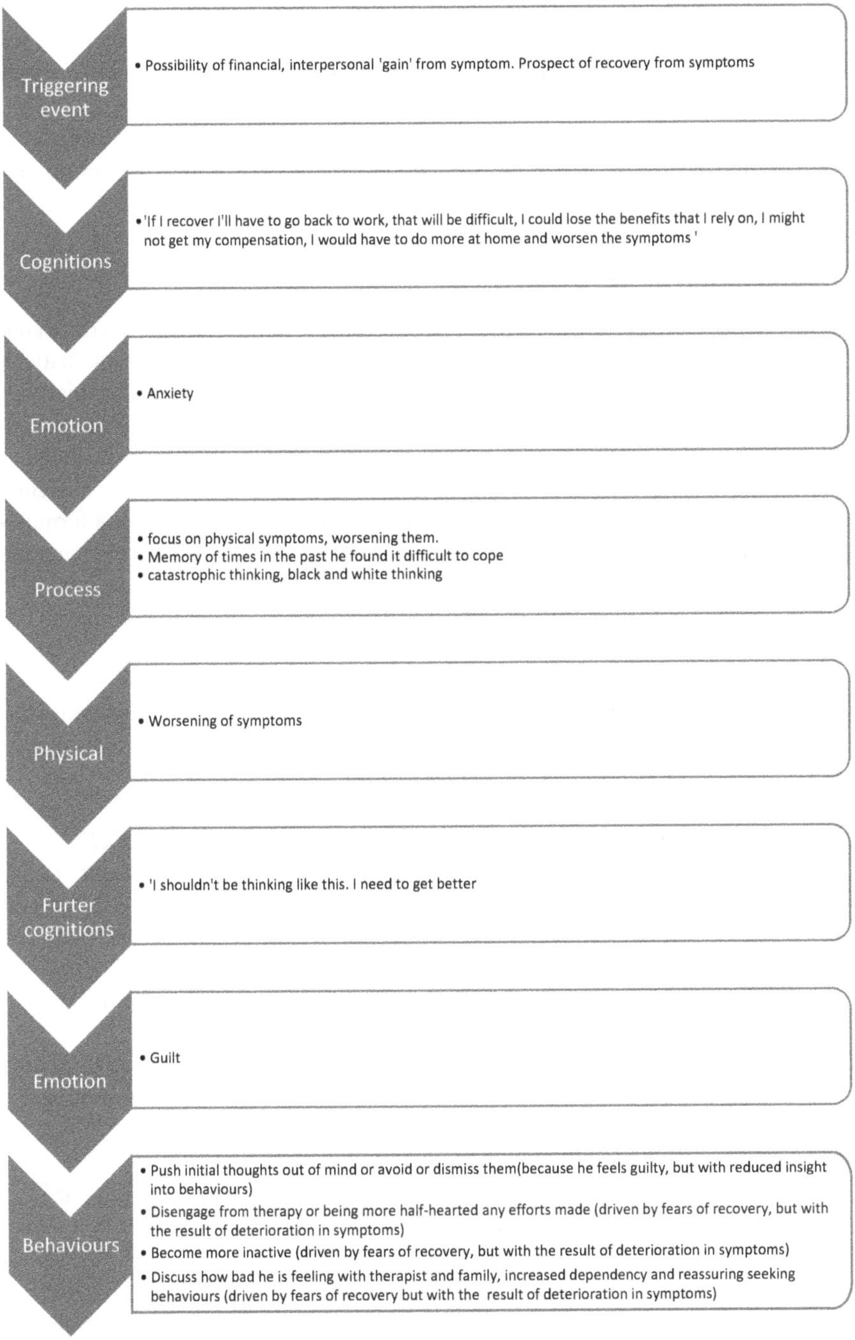

**Triggering event**

- Possibility of financial, interpersonal 'gain' from symptom. Prospect of recovery from symptoms

**Cognitions**

- 'If I recover I'll have to go back to work, that will be difficult, I could lose the benefits that I rely on, I might not get my compensation, I would have to do more at home and worsen the symptoms '

**Emotion**

- Anxiety

**Process**

- focus on physical symptoms, worsening them.
- Memory of times in the past he found it difficult to cope
- catastrophic thinking, black and white thinking

**Physical**

- Worsening of symptoms

**Furter cognitions**

- 'I shouldn't be thinking like this. I need to get better

**Emotion**

- Guilt

**Behaviours**

- Push initial thoughts out of mind or avoid or dismiss them(because he feels guilty, but with reduced insight into behaviours)
- Disengage from therapy or being more half-hearted any efforts made (driven by fears of recovery, but with the result of deterioration in symptoms)
- Become more inactive (driven by fears of recovery, but with the result of deterioration in symptoms)
- Discuss how bad he is feeling with therapist and family, increased dependency and reassuring seeking behaviours (driven by fears of recovery but with the result of deterioration in symptoms)

*Figure 14.1* Fear of recovery

- They may be expecting an insurance payout, or may be in receipt of it, and this payment is dependent on continual illness and disability
- The person's family may have been increasingly attentive and caring when the patient was ill, and there is a risk of losing this attention if recovery occurs
- They may have strong dependent traits or even dependent personality disorder
- Full recovery may lead to the discontinuation of medications such as opioids that the person has become dependent on

### Addressing fear of recovery

If there is some concern that fear of recovery is present, the therapist needs to consider what to do. The first issue is whether to share this concern with the patient, using a formulation. It is normal practice in CBT to fully share formulations; however, the danger here may be that this formulation may alienate the patient and cause them to drop out of treatment. An assessment will have to be made as to whether this sharing and collaboration is a good idea: if the patient has good insight, there is a good therapeutic relationship, then it is wise to share a formulation at least of a basic kind. Conversely, if there is a lot of resistance, anger and hostility and the general sense that the patient will be unable to contemplate a formulation that includes fear of recovery, then it will be better to hold back. The formulation needs to be shared and developed collaboratively and at a timely moment, in the context of a good therapeutic relationship; it should be some way into the therapy, and it should be done sensitively, and in a non-judgemental way. (If the formulation is not shared it can still be used by the therapist to guide their interventions). Here are some ways to approach it:

- I'm wondering if you have any anxieties about going back to work?
- Do you have any concerns at all about fully recovering from your symptoms?
- If I was in your position, I'd be concerned about losing my benefits/not getting my insurance payout. Have you got any concerns about that? Does that impede your recovery?
- Have you heard of the idea of the sick role? Do you think this applies to you at any level?
- I've noticed that as you get better, and your symptoms reduce, you seem more anxious. Is there any reason for that? Have you got any concerns about making your full recovery?
- Can I discuss a sensitive and confidential issue with you?
- Do you think that having your symptoms play some sort of role in your life?
- Is your unconscious mind telling you to hold onto your symptoms?
- Do your symptoms relate to some experience in your past?

It is important when approaching this that the therapist's tone is compassionate and objective, emphasising that this response is understandable and normal, and a stance of Socratic questioning, and guided discovery should be used. The patient's response is likely to be on a continuum from angry denial to full acceptance, and anything in between. If the dialogue is opened then pros and cons of abnormal illness behaviour can be considered in the short and long term, for example:

*T:*   It looks like we agreed that you're quite fearful of getting better.
*P:*   I'm quite anxious about going back to work, as that's where the problem started in the first place.
*T:*   What's your specific worry about going back to work?
*P:*   The symptoms that I had before, the headaches, will be worsened if I go back to work.
*T:*   How does this worry affect your response to therapy?
*P:*   I'm probably not putting the same effort in that I used to do.
*T:*   I noticed that. What are the consequences of this now and in the future, for you?
*P:*   I'm likely to be stuck with the symptoms for a while longer, but I would have longer off work.
*T:*   Can we try and work with this?

Hopefully, the patient will consider that a prolonged period of being stuck with symptoms will be worse that the possibility of returning to employment, and often there are schemes of gradual return to work that could mitigate some of their fears. Sometimes, however, one gets a sense of the reinforcers for being ill being so strong, or the fear of recovery being so powerful, that therapeutic progress can't be made. For example, if there is a very attentive spouse, a generous benefits payment, and a strong fear of going back into the old situation that triggered the symptoms, then there is little that the therapist can do to overcome this.

A possible step-by-step approach to this problem is as follows:

- Hold the full formulation back for the time being until the therapeutic relationship is stronger.
- Broaden the goals away from symptoms on to valued areas such as relationships, work and hobbies. Spend more time talking about this and focusing on this, than on symptoms.
- Gently explore cognitions and emotions around fear of recovery, and see what response there is from the patient.
- Emphasise that it is perfectly understandable if a person has a fear of recovery, but engage with the negative consequences of this in the short and longer term. Bring in ideas of resilience (Chapter 7), as the patient may be underestimating this in themselves.
- Engage with the family if they are a powerful maintenance factor, trying to agree some joint goals of encouraging independence, and self-reliance.
- Ask the person if they know of anyone else (whom they have known since childhood) who has a chronic physical condition and ask what they think of

*Table 14.1* Further strategies to address fear of recovery

| | |
|---|---|
| Insurance or financial benefits are discouraging recovery. | Emphasise that the symptoms could get stuck. Discuss this in terms of values of a healthy worthwhile life. Negotiate reduction of benefits and increase of working hours as experiment. |
| Attentive family or spouse. | Bring family into session. Negotiate patient's increased independence and reduced family attention. Increase rewards for independence. Reflect on what happened when this is done. |
| Dependent personality traits. | Understand these as unhelpful rules such as 'I can't cope by myself', or 'I need others to make decisions for me', and follow this up with behavioural experiments. |
| Dependency on opiates or benzodiazepines. | Explore fears of coming off meds. Involve a pharmacist. |
| Significant family/work demands on patient if they fully recover. | Explore worries about this with patient. Try to negotiate with work or family a gradual increase of demands. |

them, how it affected them over the years. The patient can be asked if they felt there was any 'silver lining', or any benefits from them being ill. The patient is then asked if any of this is relevant to their life. Discussion can progress to asking if the patient needs help with assertiveness, as secondary gain undermines assertiveness because it means getting something without asking (Woolfolk & Allen, 2007). If the secondary gain benefits have been identified in discussion, more constructive and helpful ways of gaining these benefits can be discussed (Woolfolk & Allen, 2007).

•   Use dialogue separating out the part of the person who wants to fully recover and the part of the person who is fearful of this: 'Is the part of you that is fearful speaking here?', 'Is the hidden fearful side coming out here', 'How is the fearful side of you behaving?' and 'What would the braver side of you say to them?'. This can be enhanced by doing empty chair exercises, dialoguing the two sides as follows. Ask the patient to consent to doing an empty chair exercise (Kellogg, 2004). The person could be asked to say (from the fearful side) why they are fearful of recovery/progress, and then swap chairs and say why it is better to recover. The patient will swap chairs until the dialogue is finished, ending on the healthy side.

If the patient is very resistant to the idea of fear of recovery, and even reacts in an angry way, there are a few possibilities. Bring the topic back in at a future date, having given the patient time to consider it. Also, keep the formulation of fear of recovery in mind as you design and implement future interventions. Another possibility is exploring a meta-cognitive perspective, trying to understand what their thoughts and feelings are about your hypothesis. One could ask 'what are you thinking about and how are you feeling, when I bring up the topic of fear of recovery, how does it affect your behaviour in the session?' Another issue is how the therapist responds to this situation, for example with thoughts like 'they're not trying hard', 'they don't want to get better', 'they're not really ill' and 'they've too much to gain' leading to emotions such as anger or irritation, and therapist behaviours such as making a weaker therapeutic effort, shortening the session and dwelling on the desire to punish the patient by discharging them. In this case, it is important to use 'CBT from the inside' (Bennett-Levy, 2019), where the therapist understands their own negative reactions and works on these, challenging their own negative thoughts and behaviours.

An alternative technique is based on a therapy called Coherence therapy, also called memory reconsolidation therapy (Ecker, Ticic & Hulley, 2012). The authors here believe that all patients have an anti-symptom position (that they don't like the symptom, it is horrible, it should go away), which is easily accessible. They also believe that patients have a pro-symptom position: this means that there is a position that holds the symptoms to be valuable or having a useful or protective function, that is rooted in the past and is not easily available to awareness. This is done by asking the patient to bring to mind an incidence of the symptom; they are then asked to consider what it would be like not to have the symptom, by gentle Socratic questioning, being aware of non-verbal communication, dwelling on symptoms, and gently exploring this. Although the initial position is anti-symptom with questioning, the pro-symptom attachment may be brought to mind. This is done by asking for a specific example and then exploring the appeal that the symptom actually has. This may be done by sentence completion, the therapist starts a sentence, for example 'if I did not have fatigue then. . .', and the patient is asked to complete it. And overt statement of the pro- and anti-symptom position is made and the patient take steps to integrate that into their life, so that the symptom is not necessary.

Example of dialogue

*T:* I just wanted to explore these symptoms through an exercise asking you to bring to mind an example of them.

*P:* Em . . . ok.

*T:* You seem a bit unsure. I'm just going to ask you about the symptoms after I've asked you to bring an example to mind.

*P:* OK then.

*T:* Can you bring to mind a specific example when your pain and fatigue particularly bad?

*P:* The one that comes to mind was having to do the exercise, the walk, that you suggested I do.

*T:* Okay that sounds tough. But bear with me and I'd like you to describe what you're thinking now, what you're feeling, what are your symptoms like when you are starting to do the walk.

Patient does this and is tearful.

*T:* Can I now ask you to finish a sentence, 'If I don't have the symptoms. . . .'

*P:* Everything would be better.

*T:* Is there anything at all that would not be better?

*P:* I'd end up doing all the things I did before, a very stressful job, having to run the house and mind the kids very much help. I guess that is something that would not be better.

*T:* That sounds tough. Maybe the symptoms have played a role in your life up to now?

*P:* Maybe

*T:* Perhaps we can look at whether you really need them.

This example is relatively straightforward and with many patients subtly and gently exploring this will be requited, and it may not be successful.

### Further specific case examples

James was 25; he had lived with his parents all his life, and had not held down a permanent job, but he had done some temporary work. He presented to me (PK) with diffuse symptoms of pain and fatigue. I identified strengths of a good sense of humour and a powerful desire to change in some direction. I did not want to present the formulation of fear of recovery, straight away, so I held this back, and focused on building a therapeutic relationship, and setting some goals. James wanted to focus entirely on symptom reduction; however I worked on broadening the goals to include value-based living in terms of working and relationships. It was a bit difficult to focus on symptoms as we struggled to find specific factors that worsened the symptoms. When I talked about moving towards his various goals such as getting a job and earning money, and developing a romantic relationship, it was met by comments about the symptoms stopping him doing this. I tried to explore this by asking questions such as 'what would you do if you didn't have the symptoms', 'In what way did the symptoms get in the way of doing this' and 'Do you think your body is generating the symptoms because it's fearful of taking the steps'. Here James was able to answer these questions thoughtfully and truthfully and gain some insight into his predicament: this allowed us to do some negative thought work on challenging his anxious predictions around moving forward. As we did so there was much less discussion of symptoms and more focus on his life, and we eventually had a considerable success in getting him into a work rehabilitation program, which he made a success of.

Julie was 30 and living with a boyfriend. Some of the warning signs of secondary gain were there at the beginning, including a history of unemployment, a very attentive and caring boyfriend, a longish period on sickness benefits, a legal claim for compensation, a confusing story of weakness and pain in her left side. In the formulation in my mind, I (PK) felt that her boyfriend was very attentive and self-sacrificing, and his personality was interacting unhelpfully with her dependent traits. Again, I tried to move to setting goals away from just symptoms and tried to build up a therapeutic relationship, but it was harder here. I felt there were rules for living in play 'If I'm ill, I won't have to face things', 'I need others to help me cope.' This led to strong traits such as focusing on symptoms, avoidance and being dependent on boyfriend, and these were out of Julie's awareness. Although I encouraged her to take steps towards her goal of getting a job, she reported a very significant increase in symptoms when she walked or exercised or did housework. After a while she seemed less engaged with therapy, and missed appointments. Her boyfriend came in for sessions as a co-therapist, but we could not get an agreed formulation; he could not accept that she was doing anything other than trying her best. I tried to discuss Julie's rules for living with her and although we agreed them to be reasonably accurate, we could not get agreement they were anything to do with her symptoms, and eventually therapy fizzled out.

If the strategies described earlier do not work and the fear of recovery factors are strong, it may be necessary to discharge the patient.

If the patient is moving to a more planned discharge, then the therapist must develop a collaborative relapse prevention or maintaining progress plan, in line with standard CBT procedure. There are various templates for this but they all ask the patient to summarise what they have learnt from the therapy, what they have changed about their thoughts and behaviours, what could cause problems in the future, what this would look like from a symptom perspective and what the patient should do to maintain progress and prevent relapse. Are there any special considerations for the long-term conditions and MUS group? There is not any research to guide this, but the main difference is that we are working with a group whose problems potentially can be chronic and difficult to treat, so the most useful phrase is probably 'maintaining progress'. With MUS there will be an emphasis on continuing to manage the maintenance factors that are contributing to the MUS, and with anxiety and depression relapse prevention would look similar to how it is done typically, with emphasis on maintaining health behaviours of facing into avoidances, but perhaps with most more emphasis on identifying physical symptoms as a trigger or manifestation of the anxiety/depression.

In concluding the book, we hope that the reader has some ideas and inspiration to help the long-term condition and MUS patients, and we wish you well in that endeavour.

## Chapter summary

Occasionally patients become fearful of recovery and this can impede progress. The research evidence would back this up, and it is sometimes called secondary gain. Factors that might show it is present are as follows: symptoms don't seem as severe as described, family are very attentive, history of dependent traits, financial benefits and confusing history. This topic needs to be brought up sensitively in the context of a good therapeutic relationship, and could be formulated. Suggestions are made as to how to introduce the topic and deal with it, with some case examples. A maintaining progress (or relapse prevention) plan should be done with all patients.

# References

Abramowitz, J. S., Deacon, B. J., & Valentiner, D. P. (2007). The Short Health Anxiety Inventory: Psychometric properties and construct validity in a non-clinical sample. *Cognitive Therapy and Research, 31*(6), 871–883.

American Psychiatric Association. (2000). *Diagnostic and statistical manual of mental disorders (DSM-4-TR ®)*. Washington DC: American Psychiatric Pub.

American Psychiatric Association. (2013). *Diagnostic and statistical manual of mental disorders (DSM-5®)*. Washington DC: American Psychiatric Pub.

Andersson, G. (2009). Using the Internet to provide cognitive behaviour therapy. *Behaviour Research and Therapy, 47*(3), 175–180.

Andrews, G., Basu, A., Cuijpers, P., Craske, M. G., McEvoy, P., English, C. L., & Newby, J. M. (2018). Computer therapy for the anxiety and depression disorders is effective, acceptable and practical health care: An updated meta-analysis. *Journal of Anxiety Disorders, 55*, 70–78.

Arntz, A. (2012). Imagery rescripting as a therapeutic technique: Review of clinical trials, basic studies, and research agenda. *Journal of Experimental Psychopathology, 3*(2), 189–208.

Atkinson, D., McCarthy, M., & Walmsley, J. (Eds.). (2000). *Good times, bad times: Women with learning difficulties telling their stories*. Kidderminster: BiLd.

Bagby, R. M., Parker, J. D., & Taylor, G. J. (1994). The twenty-item Toronto Alexithymia Scale – I. Item selection and cross-validation of the factor structure. *Journal of Psychosomatic Research, 38*(1), 23–32.

Baider, L., Uziely, B., & Kaplan De-Nour, A. (1994). Progressive muscle relaxation and guided imagery in cancer patients. *General Hospital Psychiatry, 16*(5), 340–347.

Barends, H., Claassen-van Dessel, N., van der Wouden, J. C., Twisk, J. W., Terluin, B., van der Horst, H. E., & Dekker, J. (2020). Impact of symptom focusing and somatosensory amplification on persistent physical symptoms: A three-year follow-up study. *Journal of Psychosomatic Research*, 110131.

Barker, P. (2001). The Tidal Model: Developing an empowering, person-centred approach to recovery within psychiatric and psychiatric- mental health nursing. *Journal of Psychiatric and Psychiatric Mental Health Nursing, 8*(3), 233–240.

Barrera, T. L., Grubbs, K. M., Kunik, M. E., & Teng, E. J. (2014). A review of cognitive behavioral therapy for panic disorder in patients with chronic obstructive pulmonary disease: The rationale for interoceptive exposure. *Journal of Clinical Psychology in Medical Settings, 21*(2), 144–154.

Beck, A. T. (1976). *Cognitive therapy and the emotional disorders*. New York: Madison.

Beck, A. T., Emery, G., & Greenberg, R. L. (1985). *Anxiety disorders and phobias*. New York: Basic Books.

Beck, A. T., Emery, G., & Greenberg, R. L. (2005). *Anxiety disorders and phobias: A cognitive perspective*. New York: Basic Books.

Beck, A. T., Rush, J., Shaw, B., & Emery, G. (1979). *Cognitive therapy of depression*. New York: Guilford Press.

Bennett-Levy, J. E. (2019). Why therapists should walk the talk: The theoretical and empirical case for personal practice in therapist training and professional development. *Journal of Behavior Therapy and Experimental Psychiatry, 62*, 133–145.

Bennett-Levy, J. E., Butler, G. E., Fennell, M. E., Hackman, A. E., Mueller, M. E., & Westbrook, D. E. (2004). *Oxford guide to behavioural experiments in cognitive therapy*. Oxford: Oxford University Press.

Bennett-Levy, J. E., Thwaites, R., Haarhoff, B., & Perry, H. (2015). *Self-practice/self-reflection guides for psychotherapists. Experiencing CBT from the inside out: A self-practice/self-reflection workbook for therapists*. New York: Guilford Press.

Benton, T., Staab, J., & Evans, D. L. (2007). Medical co-morbidity in depressive disorders. *Annals of Clinical Psychiatry, 19*(4), 289–303.

Beresnevaite, M. (2000). Exploring the benefits of group psychotherapy in reducing alexithymia in coronary heart disease patients: A preliminary study. *Psychotherapy and Psychosomatics, 69*(3), 117–122.

Bilotta, E., Giacomantonio, M., Leone, L., Mancini, F., & Coriale, G. (2016). Being alexithymic: Necessity or convenience. Negative emotionality × avoidant coping interactions and alexithymia. *Psychology and Psychotherapy: Theory, Research and Practice, 89*(3), 261–275.

Blackwell, S. E., Rius-Ottenheim, N., Schulte-van Maaren, Y. W. M., Carlier, I. V. E., Middelkoop, V. D., Zitman, F. G., . . . Giltay, E. J. (2013). Optimism and mental imagery: A possible cognitive marker to promote wellbeing? *Psychiatry Research, 206*, 56–61.

Bonvanie, I. J., Janssens, K. A., Rosmalen, J. G., & Oldehinkel, A. J. (2017). Life events and functional somatic symptoms: A population study in older adolescents. *British Journal of Psychology, 108*(2), 318–333.

Borkovec, T. D. (1985). Worry: A potentially valuable concept. *Behaviour Research and Therapy, 23*, 481–482.

Borkovec, T. D., Robinson, E., Pruzinsky, T., & DePree, J. A. (1983). Preliminary exploration of worry: Some characteristics and processes. *Behaviour Research and Therapy, 21*, 9–16.

Borkovec, T. D., Shadick, R. N., & Hopkins, M. (1991). The nature of normal and pathological worry. In R. M. Rapee & D. H. Barlow (Eds.), *Chronic anxiety: Generalized anxiety disorder and mixed anxiety-depression*. New York: Guilford Press.

Brewin, C. R. (2006). Understanding cognitive-behaviour therapy: A retrieval competition account. *Behaviour Research and Therapy, 44*, 765–784.

Brewin, C. R., Wheatley, J., Patel, T., Fearon, P., Hackman, A, Wells, A., . . Myers, S. (2009). Imagery rescripting as a brief stand-alone treatment for depressed patients with intrusive memories. *Behaviour Research and Therapy, 47*(7), 569–576.

Brown, R. J. (2004). Psychological mechanisms of medically unexplained symptoms: An integrative conceptual model. *Psychological Bulletin, 130*(5), 793.

Burns, D. D. (2012). *Feeling good*. New York: Harper Books.

Butler, G., & Surawy, C. (2004). Avoidance of affect. *Oxford Guide to Behavioural Experiments in Cognitive Therapy*, *2*, 351.

Carlsson, A. M. (1983). Assessment of chronic pain. I. Aspects of the reliability and validity of the visual analogue scale. *Pain*, *16*(1), 87–101.

Carter, T., Morres, I. D., Meade, O., & Callaghan, P. (2016). The effect of exercise on depressive symptoms in adolescents: A systematic review and meta-analysis. *Journal of the American Academy for Child and Adolescent Psychiatry*, *55*(7), 580–590.

Chalder, T. (1995). *Overcoming Chronic Fatigue*. London: Robinson.

Chalder, T., Berelowitz, G., Pawlikowska, T., Watts, L., Wessely, S., Wright, D., & Wallace, E. P. (1993). Development of a fatigue scale. *Journal of Psychosomatic Research*, *37*(2), 147–153.

Chalder, T., & Willis, C. (2017). 'Lumping' and 'splitting' medically unexplained symptoms: Is there a role for a transdiagnostic approach? *Journal of Mental Health*, *26*(3), 187–191.

Chalder, T., Windgassen, S. S., Sibelli, A., Burgess, M., & Moss-Morris, R. (2014*). Regul8: A self-management programme for IBS*. London: NHS Health Education England.

Charis, C., & Panayiotou, G. (Eds.). (2018). *Somatoform and other psychosomatic disorders: A dialogue between contemporary psychodynamic psychotherapy and cognitive behavioral therapy perspectives*. New York: Springer.

Cheatle, M. D., Foster, S., Pinkett, A., Lesneski, M., Qu, D., & Dhingra, L. (2016). Assessing and managing sleep disturbance in patients with chronic pain. *Anesthesiology Clinics*, *34*(2), 379–393.

Chellingsworth, M. (2020a). *Get back to being you with Behavioural Activation (BA) protocol: Clinician's guide*. Exeter: The CBT Resource.

Chellingsworth, M. (2020b). *Fears conquered with exposure and habituation protocol: A clinician's guide*. Exeter: The CBT Resource.

Chellingsworth, M. (2020c). *Live more worry less with GAD protocol: A clinician's guide*. Exeter: The CBT Resource.

Chew-Graham, C. A., Dowrick, C., Wearden, A., Richardson, V., & Peters, S. (2010). Making the diagnosis of chronic fatigue syndrome/myalgic encephalitis in primary care: A qualitative study. *BMC Family Practice*, *11*(1), 16.

Chew-Graham, C. A., Heyland, S., Kingstone, T., Shepherd, T., Buszewicz, M., Burroughs, H., & Sumathipala, A. (2017). Medically unexplained symptoms: Continuing challenges for primary care. *British Journal of General Practice*, *67*(656), 106–107.

Chikersal, P., Belgrave, D., Dohety, G., Enrique, A., Palacios, J. E., Richards, D., & Thieme, A. (2020, April 25–30). Understanding client support strategies to improve clinical outcomes in an online mental health intervention. *CHI'20*, 2020, Honolulu, HI, USA.

Clarke, A., Hanson, E., & Ross, H. (2003). Seeing the person behind the patient: Enhancing the care of older people using a biographical approach. *Journal of Clinical Nursing*, *12*(2), 697–706.

Clarke, D. M., & Currie, K. C. (2009). Depression, anxiety, and their relationship with chronic diseases: A review of the epidemiology, risk, and treatment evidence. *Medical Journal of Australia*, *190*, S54–S60.

Cleare, A. J. (2004). The HPA axis and the genesis of chronic fatigue syndrome. *Trends in Endocrinology & Metabolism*, *15*(2), 55–59.

Constantinou, E. (2018). Negative affect and medically unexplained symptoms. In *Somatoform and other psychosomatic disorders* (pp. 61–87). Cham: Springer.

Contrada, R., & Baum, A. (Eds.). (2010). *The handbook of stress science: Biology, psychology, and health*. New York: Springer.

Conwell, Y., Duberstein, P. R., & Caine, E. D. (2002). Risk factors for suicide in later life. *Biological Psychiatry*, *52*(3), 193–204.

Cook, R., Brewer, R., Shah, P., & Bird, G. (2013). Alexithymia, not autism, predicts poor recognition of emotional facial expressions. *Psychological Science*, *24*(5), 723–732.

Cooper, K., Gregory, J. D., Walker, I., Lambe, S., & Salkovskis, P. M. (2017). Cognitive behaviour therapy for health anxiety: A systematic review and meta-analysis. *Behavioural and Cognitive Psychotherapy*, *45*(2), 110–123.

Cordova, M. J., Riba, M. B., & Spiegel, D. (2017). Post-traumatic stress disorder and cancer. *The Lancet Psychiatry*, *4*(4), 330–338.

Craig, T. K. J., Drake, H., Mills, K., & Boardman, A. P. (1994). The South London Somatisation Study: II. Influence of stressful life events, and secondary gain. *The British Journal of Psychiatry*, *165*(2), 248–258.

Crane, C., Shah, D., Barnhofer, T., & Holmes, E. A. (2012). Suicidal imagery in a previously depressed community sample. *Clinical Psychology and Psycho-therapy*, *19*, 57–69.

Craske, M. G., Hermans, D., & Vervliet, B. (2018). State-of-the-art and future directions for extinction as a translational model for fear and anxiety. *Philosophical Transactions of the Royal Society B: Biological Sciences*, *373*(1742), 20170025.

Creed, F. H., Tomenson, B., Chew-Graham, C., Macfarlane, G. J., Davies, I., Jackson, J., . . . McBeth, J. (2013). Multiple somatic symptoms predict impaired health status in functional somatic syndromes. *International Journal of Behavioral Medicine*, *20*(2), 194–205.

Cruwys, T., Wakefield, J. R. H., Sani, F., Dingle, G. A., & Jetten, J. (2018). A doctor a day keeps loneliness at bay? Social isolation, health status, and frequent attendance in primary care. *Annals of Behavioural Medicine*, *52*(10), 817–829.

Culpepper, L. (2009). Generalized anxiety disorder and medical illness. *The Journal of Clinical Psychiatry*, *70*(suppl 2), 20–24.

Currie, S. R., Wilson, K. G., & Curran, D. (2002). Clinical significance and predictors of treatment response to cognitive-behavior therapy for insomnia secondary to chronic pain. *Journal of Behavioral Medicine*, *25*(2), 135–153.

Daniels, N. F., Ridwan, R., Barnard, E. B., Amanullah, T. M., & Hayhurst, C. (2021). A comparison of emergency Department presentations for medically unexplained symptoms in frequent attenders during COVID-19. *Clinical Medicine.* Published pre-print on May 20, 2021 as doi:10.7861/clinmed.2020-1093

Deary, V., Chalder, T., & Sharpe, M. (2007). The cognitive behavioural model of medically unexplained symptoms: A theoretical and empirical review. *Clinical Psychology Review*, *27*(7), 781–797.

De Gucht, V. (2003). Stability of neuroticism and alexithymia in somatization. *Comprehensive Psychiatry*, *44*(6), 466–471.

Department of Health. (2011). *Talking therapies: A four-year plan of action.* A supporting document to No Health without Mental Health policy paper.

Department of Health. (2015). *2010–2015 Government policy long term health conditions.* London: UK Stationery Office.

Deshmukh, V. M., Toelle, B. G., Usherwood, T., O'Grady, B., & Jenkins, C. R. (2007). Anxiety, panic, and adult asthma: A cognitive-behavioral perspective. *Respiratory Medicine*, *101*(2), 194–202.

Dimitrov, L., Moschopoulou, E., & Korszun, A. (2019). Interventions for the treatment of cancer-related traumatic stress symptoms: A systematic review of the literature. *Psycho-oncology*, *28*(5), 970–979.

Dowell, D., Haegerich, T. M., & Chou, R. (2016). CDC guideline for prescribing opioids for chronic pain – United States, 2016. *JAMA, 315*(15), 1624–1645.

Driessen, E., & Hollon, S. D. (2010). Cognitive behavioral therapy for mood disorders: Efficacy, moderators and mediators. *The Psychiatric Clinics of North America, 33*(3), 537–555.

Druss, B., & Pincus, H. (2000). Suicidal ideation and suicide attempts in general medical illnesses. *Archives of Internal Medicine, 160*(10), 1522–1526.

Dugas, M. J., & Robichaud, M. (2007). *Practical clinical guidebooks. Cognitive-behavioral treatment for generalized anxiety disorder: From science to practice.* Oxford: Routledge/Taylor & Francis Group.

Dunkel-Schetter, C., Feinstein, L. G., Taylor, S. E., & Falke, R. L. (1992). Patterns of coping with cancer. *Health Psychology, 11*(2), 79–87.

Dworkin, R. H., Turk, D. C., Revicki, D. A., Harding, G., Coyne, K. S., Peirce-Sandner, S., . . . Farrar, J. T. (2009). Development and initial validation of an expanded and revised version of the Short-form McGill Pain Questionnaire (SF-MPQ-2). *PAIN®, 144*(1–2), 35–42.

D'Zurilla, T. J., & Nezu, A. M. (1982). Social problem solving in adults. In P. C. Kendall (Ed.), *Advances in cognitive-behavioral research and therapy* (Vol. 1, pp. 201–274). New York: Academic Press.

D'Zurilla, T. J., & Nezu, A. M. (2010). Problem-solving therapy. *Handbook of Cognitive-Behavioral Therapies, 3*, 197–225.

Eaton, W. W., Martins, S. S., Nestadt, G., Bienvenu, O. J., Clarke, D., & Alexandre, P. (2008). The burden of mental disorders. *Epidemiologic Reviews, 30*(1), 1–14.

Ecker, B., Ticic, R., & Hulley, L. (2012). *Unlocking the emotional brain: Eliminating symptoms at their roots using memory reconsolidation.* Oxford: Routledge.

Ehlers, A., & Clark, D. M. (2000). A cognitive model of posttraumatic stress disorder. *Behaviour Research and Therapy, 38*(4), 319–345.

Ekers, D., Richards, D., & Gilbody, S. (2008). A meta-analysis of behavioural therapy for depression. *Psychological Medicine, 38*, 611–623.

Factor, S. A., Podskalny, G. D., & Molho, E. S. (1995). Psychogenic movement disorders: Frequency, clinical profile, and characteristics. *Journal of Neurology, Neurosurgery & Psychiatry, 59*(4), 406–412.

Farrand, P. (Ed.). (2020). *Low Intensity CBT Skills and Interventions: A practitioner's manual.* Exeter: Sage.

Feifel, H., Strack, S., & Nagy, V. T. (1987). Coping strategies and associated features of medically ill patients. *Psychosomatic Medicine, 49*(6), 616–625.

Fennell, M. (1999). *Overcoming low self-esteem.* London: Robinson.

Ferster, C. B. (1973). A functional analysis of depression. *American Psychologist, 28*, 857–870.

Fink, P., & Schröder, A. (2010). One single diagnosis, bodily distress syndrome, succeeded to capture 10 diagnostic categories of functional somatic syndromes and somatoform disorders. *Journal of Psychosomatic Research, 68*, 415–426.

Fishbain, D. A., Rosomoff, H. L., Cutler, R. B., & Rosomoff, R. S. (1995). Secondary gain concept: A review of the scientific evidence. *The Clinical Journal of Pain, 11*(1), 6–21.

Fitzpatrick, S. L., Schumann, K. P., & Hill-Briggs, F. (2013). Problem-solving interventions for diabetes self-management and control: A systematic review of literature. *Diabetes Research & Clinical Practice, 100*(2), 145–161.

Fleet, R. P., & Beitman, B. D. (1998). Cardiovascular death from panic disorder and panic-like anxiety: A critical review of the literature. *Journal of Psychosomatic Research, 44*(1), 71–80.

Fletcher, G. F., Landolfo, C., Niebauer, J., Ozemek, C., Arena, R., & Lavie, C. J. (2018). Promoting physical activity and exercise: JACC health promotion series. *Journal of the American College of Cardiology, 72*(14), 1622–1639.

Francis, C. Y., Morris, J., & Whorwell, P. J. (1997). The irritable bowel severity scoring system: A simple method of monitoring irritable bowel syndrome and its progress. *Alimentary Pharmacology & Therapeutics, 11*(2), 395–402.

Gellatly, J., Bower, P., Hennessy, S., Richards, D., Gilbody, S., & Lovell, K. (2007). What makes self-help interventions effective in the management of depressive symptoms? Meta-analysis and meta-regression. *Psychological Medicine, 37*(9), 1217–1228.

Germer, C. K., & Chan, C. S. (2014). Mindfulness: It's not what you think. In N. Thoma & D. McKay (Eds.), *Working with emotion in cognitive behavioral therapy: Techniques for clinical practice* (pp. 11–31). New York: Guilford Press.

Gilbert, P. (2005). *Compassion: Conceptualisations, research and use in psychotherapy.* Hove: Routledge.

Gilbert, P. (2010). An introduction to compassion focused therapy in cognitive behavior therapy. *International Journal of Cognitive Therapy, 3*, 97–112.

Goldstein, L. H., Robinson, E. J., Mellers, J. D., Stone, J., Carson, A., Reuber, M., . . . Pilecka, I. (2020). Cognitive behavioural therapy for adults with dissociative seizures (CODES): A pragmatic, multicentre, randomised controlled trial. *The Lancet Psychiatry, 7*(6), 491–505.

Goldstein, L. H., Robinson, E. J., Reuber, M., Chalder, T., Callaghan, H., Eastwood, C., . . . Moore, M. (2019). Characteristics of 698 patients with dissociative seizures: A UK multi-center study. *Epilepsia, 60*(11), 2182–2193.

Graham, C. D., Gouick, J., Krahe, C., & Gillanders, D. (2016). A systematic review of the use of acceptance and commitment therapy (ACT) in chronic disease and long-term conditions. *Clinical Psychology Review, 46*, 46–58.

Greco, M. (2012). The classification and nomenclature of 'medically unexplained symptoms': Conflict, performativity and critique. *Social Science & Medicine, 75*(12), 2362–2369.

Green, J., Tones, K., Cross, R., & Woodall, J. (2015). *Health promotion: Planning and strategies.* Los Angeles: Sage.

Greenberger, D., & Padesky, C. A. (2015). *Mind over mood: Change how you feel by changing the way you think.* New York: Guilford Press.

Greer, S., Moorey, S., Baruch, J. D., Watson, M., Robertson, B. M., Mason, A., . . . Bliss, J. M. (1992). Adjuvant psychological therapy for patients with cancer: A prospective randomised trial. *BMJ, 304*(6828), 675–680.

Gruber, J., Prinstein, M. J., Clark, L. A., Rottenberg, J., Abramowitz, J. S., Albano, A. M., . . . Weinstock, L. M. (2020). Mental health and clinical psychological science in the time of COVID-19: Challenges, opportunities, and a call to action. *American Psychologist, 76*(3), 409–426.

Grünewald, R. (2019). What are non-epileptic seizures, and why do people have them? *British Journal of Hospital Medicine, 80*(11), 652–657.

Guest, J. (2015). *The CBT art activity book: 100 illustrated handouts for therapeutic work.* London: Jessica Kingsley Publishers.

Guest, J. (2020). *The CBT art workbook for managing stress*. London: Jessica Kingsley Publishers.

Haddad, M. (2009). Depression in adults with a chronic physical health problem: Treatment and management. *International Journal of Nursing Studies, 46*, 1411–1414.

Hadert, A. (2013). *Adapting guided self-help for people with long-term conditions* (Unpublished thesis). Doctorate in Clinical Psychology, University of Exeter.

Harwood, J., & Sparks, L. (2003). Social identity and health: An intergroup communication approach to cancer. *Health Communication, 15*, 145–159.

Haslam, C., Cruwys, T., Haslam, S. A., Bentley, S. V., Dingle, G. A., & Chang, M. X.-L. (2016c). Groups 4 health: Evidence that a social identity intervention that builds and strengthens social group membership improves mental health. *Journal of Affective Disorders, 194*, 188–195.

Haslam, C., Cruwys, T., Haslam, S. A., Bentley, S. V., Dingle, G. A., & Jetten, J. (2016a). *GROUPS4HEALTH manual (version 3.0) Social identities and Groups Network (SIGN)*. Brisbane, Australia: University of Queensland.

Haslam, C., Cruwys, T., Haslam, S. A., Bentley, S. V., Dingle, G. A., & Jetten, J. (2016b). *GROUPS4HEALTH workbook (version 3.0) Social identities and Groups Network (SIGN)*. Brisbane, Australia: University of Queensland.

Haslam, C., Jetten, J., Cruwys, T., Dingle, G., & Haslam, S. A. (2018). *The new psychology of health: Unlocking the social cure*. Oxon: Routledge.

Haslam, S. A., O'Brien, A., Jetten, J., Vormedal, K., & Penna, S. (2005). Taking the strain: Social identity, social support, and the experience of stress. *British Journal of Social Psychology, 44*(3), 355–370.

Hatcher, S., & House, A. (2003). Life events, difficulties, and dilemmas in the onset of chronic fatigue syndrome: A case–control study. *Psychological Medicine, 33*(7), 1185–1192.

Hayes, S. C. (2004). Acceptance and commitment therapy, relational frame theory, and the third wave of behavioral and cognitive therapies. *Behavior Therapy, 35*, 639–665.

Hayes, S. C., Strosahl K., & Wilson, K. (2011). *Acceptance and commitment therapy*. London, New York: Guilford Press.

Henningsen, P., Zipfel, S., & Herzog, W. (2007). Management of functional somatic syndromes. *Lancet, 369*(9565), 946–955.

Henningsen, P., Zipfel, S., Sattel, H., & Creed, F. (2018). Management of functional somatic syndromes and bodily distress. *Psychotherapy and Psychosomatics, 87*(1), 12–31.

Hewitt, H. (2003). Tell it like it is. *Learning Disability Practice, 6*(8), 18–22.

Hewitt, H. (2006a). Uncovering identities: The role of life story work in person-centred planning. In M. Jukes & J. Aldridge (Eds.), *Person-centred practices: A therapeutic perspective*. London: Quay Books.

Hewitt, H. (2006b). *Life story books for people with learning disabilities: A practical guide*. Kidderminster: BiLd.

Hitcham, M. (2007). Life story work with children with life-threatening illnesses. In T. Ryan & R. Walker (Eds.), *Life story work: A practical guide to helping children understand their past*. London: British association for adoption and fostering.

Holmes, E. A., Crane, C., Fennell, M. J., & Williams, J. M. G. (2007). Imagery about suicide in depression – "Flash-forwards"? *Journal of Behavior Therapy and Experimental Psychiatry, 38*(4), 423–434.

Holt-Lundstad, J., Robles, T. F., & Sbarra, D. A. (2017). Advancing social connection as a public health priority in the United States. *American Psychologist, 72*, 517–530.

Hopko, D. R., Armento, M. E., Robertson, S. M., Ryba, M. M., Carvalho, J. P., Colman, J. P., et al. (2011). Brief behavioral activation and problem-solving therapy for depressed breast cancer patients: Randomized trial. *Journal of Consulting & Clinical Psychology, 79*(6), 834–849.

Hopko, D. R., Cannity, K., McIndoo, C. C., File, A. A., Ryba, M. M., Clark, C. G., et al. (2015). Behavior therapy for depressed breast cancer patients: Predictors of treatment outcome. *Journal of Consulting and Clinical Psychology, 83*(1), 225–231.

Hopko, D. R., Robertson, S. M. C., & Carvalho, J. P. (2009). Sudden gains in depressed cancer patients treated with behavioral activation therapy. *Behavior Therapy, 40*, 346–356.

Hotopf, M. (2003). Commentary on Bode et al., recurrent abdominal pain in children. *Journal of Psychosomatic Research, 54*, 423–424.

Hotopf, M. (2004). Preventing somatisation. *Psychological Medicine, 34*(2), 195–198.

Houwen, J., Lucassen, P. L., Stappers, H. W., Assendelft, P. J., & van Dulmen, S. (2017). Medically unexplained symptoms: The person, the symptoms, and the dialogue. *Family Practice, 34*(2), 245–251.

Hughes, C., Herron, S., & Younge, J. (2014). *CBT for mild to moderate depression and anxiety: A guide to low-intensity interventions.* Milton Keynes: Open University Press.

Hunt, M. G. (2016). *Reclaim your life from IBS.* New York: Sterling.

Hunt, M. G., Ertel, E., Coello, J. A., & Rodriguez, L. (2015). Empirical support for a self-help treatment for IBS. *Cognitive Therapy and Research, 39*, 215–227.

Husak, A. J., & Bair, M. J. (2020). Chronic pain and sleep disturbances: A pragmatic review of their relationships, comorbidities, and treatments. *Pain Medicine, 21*(6), 1142–1152.

IAPT. (2017). *National curriculum for psychological wellbeing practitioners to deliver low intensity interventions in the context of long-term persistent and distressing health conditions.* London: Health Education England.

Jacob, G. A., Arendt, J., Kolley, L., Scheel, C. N., Bader, K., Lieb, K., . . . Tüscher, O. (2011). Comparison of different strategies to decrease negative affect and increase positive affect in women with borderline personality disorder. *Behaviour Research and Therapy, 49*, 68–73.

Jacobson, N. S., Dobson, K. S., Truax, P. A., Addis, M. E., Koerner, K., Gollan, J. K., . . . Prince, S. E. (1996). A component analysis of cognitive-behavioral treatment for depression. *Journal of Consulting and Clinical Psychology, 64*(2), 295.

Jadhakhan, F., Lindner, O. C., Blakemore, A., & Guthrie, E. (2019). Prevalence of medically unexplained symptoms in adults who are high users of health care services: A systematic review and meta-analysis protocol. *BMJ Open, 9*(7), e027922.

Jones, C. (2010). Post-traumatic stress disorder in ICU survivors. *Journal of the Intensive Care Society, 11*(suppl 2), 12–14.

Jungmann, S. M., & Witthöft, M. (2020). Health anxiety, cyberchondria, and coping in the current COVID-19 pandemic: Which factors are related to coronavirus anxiety? *Journal of Anxiety Disorders, 73*, 102239.

Kabat-Zinn, J. (1994). *Wherever you go, there you are: Mindfulness meditation in everyday life.* New York: Hyperion.

Kangas, M., Henry, J. L., & Bryant, R. A. (2002). Posttraumatic stress disorder following cancer: A conceptual and empirical review. *Clinical Psychology Review, 22*(4), 499–524.

Kangas, M., Milross, C., & Bryant, R. A. (2014). A brief, early cognitive-behavioral program for cancer-related PTSD, anxiety, and comorbid depression. *Cognitive and Behavioral Practice, 21*(4), 416–431.

Kanzler, K. E., Bryan, C. J., McGeary, D. D., & Morrow, C. E. (2012). Suicidal ideation and perceived burdensomeness in patients with chronic pain. *Pain Practice, 12*(8), 602–609.

Katon, W. J., Richardson, L., Lozano, P., & McCauley, E. (2004). The relationship of asthma and anxiety disorders. *Psychosomatic Medicine, 66*(3), 349–355.

Kellogg, S. (2004). Dialogical encounters: Contemporary perspectives on 'Chairwork' in psychotherapy. *Psychotherapy: Theory, Research, Practice, Training, 41*(3), 310.

Kennedy, F., & Pearson, D. (2017). *Get your life back: The most effective therapies for a better you.* London: Robinson.

Kent, C., & McMillan, G. (2009). A CBT-based approach to medically unexplained symptoms. *Advances in Psychiatric Treatment, 15*(2), 146–151.

Kinsella, P. (2001). Factitious disorder: A cognitive behavioural perspective. *Behavioural and Cognitive Psychotherapy, 29*(2), 195.

Kirmayer, L. J. (1999). Rhetorics of the body: Medically unexplained symptoms in sociocultural perspective. In Y. Onoe, A. Janca, M. Asai, & N. Sartorious (Eds.), *Somatoform disorders: A world-wide perspective* (pp. 271–286). Tokyo: Springer.

Kirmayer, L. J., Groleau, D., Looper, K. J., & Dao, M. D. (2004). Explaining medically unexplained symptoms. *The Canadian Journal of Psychiatry, 49*(10), 663–672.

Kirmayer, L. J., & Taillefer, S. (1997). Somatoform disorders. In S. M. Turner & M. Hersen (Eds.), *Adult psychopathology and diagnosis* (pp. 333–383). New York: Wiley.

Klein, J. P., Berger, T., Schroder, J., Spath, C., Meyer, B., Caspar, F., . . . Moritz, S. (2013). The EVID-ENT-trial: Protocol and rationale of a multi-center randomized controlled trial testing the effectiveness of an online-based psychological intervention. *BMC Psychiatry, 13*, 239.

Kleinstäuber, M., Allwang, C., Bailer, J., Berking, M., Brünahl, C., Erkic, M., . . . Hermann, A. (2019). Cognitive behaviour therapy complemented with emotion regulation training for patients with persistent physical symptoms: A randomised clinical trial. *Psychotherapy and Psychosomatics, 88*(5), 287–299.

Kleinstäuber, M., Witthöft, M., Steffanowski, A., Van Marwijk, H. W., Hiller, W., & Lambert, M. J. (2015). Pharmacological interventions for somatoform disorders in adults, a Cochrane systematic review. *Journal of Psychosomatic Research, 6*(78), 606–607.

Kroenke, K., & Spitzer, R. L. (2002). The PHQ-9: A new depression diagnostic and severity measure. *Psychiatric Annals, 32*(9), 509–515.

Kuyken, W., Padesky, C., & Dudley, R. (2008). The science and practice of case conceptualization. *Behavioural and Cognitive Psychotherapy, 36*, 757–768.

La Forge, R. G., Rossi, J. S., Prochaska, J. O., Velicer, W. F., Levesque, V. A., & McHorney, C. A. (1999). Stage of regular exercise and health-related quality of life. *Preventive Medicine, 28*(4), 349–360.

Lane, D., Carroll, D., Ring, C., Beevers, D. G., & Lip, G. Y. (2002). The prevalence and persistence of depression and anxiety following myocardial infarction. *British Journal of Health Psychology, 7*(1), 11–21.

Larsen, J. K., Brand, N., Bermond, B., & Hijman, R. (2003). Cognitive and emotional characteristics of alexithymia: A review of neurobiological studies. *Journal of Psychosomatic Research, 54*(6), 533–541.

Lewinsohn, P. M., & Shaffer, M. (1971). The use of home observations as an integral part in the treatment of depression: Preliminary report and case studies. *Journal of Consulting and Clinical Psychology, 37*(1), 87–94.

Lewis, H. (2013). An exploratory study of primary-care therapists' perceived competence in providing cognitive behavioural therapy to people with medically unexplained symptoms. *The Cognitive Behaviour Therapist, 6.*

Lieberman, M. D., Inagaki, T. K., Tabibnia, G., & Crockett, M. J. (2011). Subjective responses to emotional stimuli during labeling, reappraisal, and distraction. *Emotion, 11*(3), 468.

Liu, J., Gill, N. S., Teodorczuk, A., Li, Z. J., & Sun, J. (2018). The efficacy of cognitive behavioural therapy in somatoform disorders and medically unexplained physical symptoms: A meta-analysis of randomized controlled trials. *Journal of Affective Disorders, 245*, 98–112.

Livermore, N., Sharpe, L., & McKenzie, D. (2010). Panic attacks and panic disorder in chronic obstructive pulmonary disease: A cognitive behavioral perspective. *Respiratory Medicine, 104*(9), 1246–1253.

Longmore, R. J., & Worrell, M. (2007). Do we need to challenge thoughts in cognitive behavior therapy?. *Clinical Psychology Review, 27*(2), 173–187.

Luminet, O., Rimé, B., Bagby, R. M., & Taylor, G. (2004). A multimodal investigation of emotional responding in alexithymia. *Cognition and Emotion, 18*(6), 741–766.

Lumley, M. A., Neely, L. C., & Burger, A. J. (2007). The assessment of alexithymia in medical settings: Implications for understanding and treating health problems. *Journal of Personality Assessment, 89*(3), 230–246.

Malouff, J. M., Thorsteinsson, E. B., & Schutte, N. S. (2007). The efficacy of problem-solving therapy in reducing mental and physical health problems: A meta-analysis. *Clinical Psychology Review, 27*(1), 46–57.

Marks, E. M., Chambers, J. B., Russell, V., & Hunter, M. S. (2016). A novel biopsychosocial, cognitive behavioural, stepped care intervention for patients with non-cardiac chest pain. *Health Psychology and Behavioral Medicine, 4*(1), 15–28.

Marks, E. M., & Hunter, S. (2015). Medically unexplained symptoms: An acceptable term? *British Journal of Pain, 9*(2), 109–114.

Marsh, A., Eslick, E. M., & Eslick, G. D. (2016). Does a diet low in FODMAPs reduce symptoms associated with functional gastrointestinal disorders? A comprehensive systematic review and meta-analysis. *European Journal of Nutrition, 55*(3), 897–906.

Masi, C. M., Chen, H.-Y., Hawkley, L. C., & Cacioppo, J. T. (2011). A meta-analysis of interventions to reduce loneliness. *Personality and Social Psychology Review, 15*, 219–266.

Masterson, C., Ekers, D., Gilbody, S., Richards, D., Toner-Clewes, B., & McMillian, D. (2014). Sudden gains in behavioural activation for depression. *Behaviour Research and Therapy, 60*, 34–38.

Mathers, N., Jones, N., & Hannay, D. (1995). Heartsink patients: A study of their general practitioners. *The British Journal of General Practice: The Journal of the Royal College of General Practitioners, 45*, 293–296.

Mathews, A., & Macleod, C. (1985). Selective processing of threat cues in anxiety states. *Behaviour Research and Therapy, 23*(5), 563–569.

Mattila, A. K., Kronholm, E., Jula, A., Salminen, J. K., Koivisto, A. M., Mielonen, R. L., & Joukamaa, M. (2008). Alexithymia and somatization in general population. *Psychosomatic Medicine, 70*(6), 716–722.

McCrae, N., Correa, A., Chan, T., Jones, S., & de Lusignan, S. (2015). Long-term conditions and medically-unexplained symptoms: feasibility of cognitive behavioural interventions within the Improving Access to Psychological Therapies Programme. *Journal of Mental Health, 24*(6), 379-384.

McEwen, B. S. (1998). Stress, adaptation, and disease: Allostasis and allostatic load. *Annals of the New York Academy of Sciences, 840*(1), 33–44.

McKeown, J., Clarke, A., & Repper, J. (2006). Life story work in health and social care: Systematic literature review. *Journal of Advanced Nursing, 55*(2), 237–247.

McLenon, J., & Rogers, M. A. (2019). The fear of needles: A systematic review and meta-analysis. *Journal of Advanced Nursing, 75*(1), 30–42.

McManus, F., Muse, K., Surwy, C., Hackman, A., & Williams, M. G. (2015). Relating differently to intrusive images: The impact of Mindfulness Based Cognitive Therapy (MBCT) on intrusive images in patients with severe health anxiety (hypochondriasis). *Mindfulness, 6*, 788–796.

Merten, T., Kaminski, A., & Pfeiffer, W. (2019). Prevalence of overreporting on symptom validity tests in a large sample of psychosomatic rehabilitation inpatients. *The Clinical Neuropsychologist*, 1–21.

Mitchell, P. H., Becker, K. J., Buzaitis, A., Cain, K. C., Fruin, M., & Kohen, R. (2008). Brief psychosocial/behavioral intervention with antidepressant reduces post-stroke depression significantly more than antidepressant alone. *Stroke, 39*(2), 543.

Mooney, K. A., & Padesky, C. (2000). Applying client creativity to recurrent problems: Constructing possibilities and tolerating doubt. *Journal of Cognitive Psychotherapy: An International Quarterly, 14*(2), 149–161.

Moreno, C., Wykes, T., Galderisi, S., Nordentoft, M., Crossley, N., Jones, N., . . . Chen, E. Y. (2020). How mental health care should change as a consequence of the COVID-19 pandemic. *The Lancet Psychiatry, 7*(9), 813–824.

Morin, C. M., Gibson, D., & Wade, J. (1998). Self-reported sleep and mood disturbance in chronic pain patients. *The Clinical Journal of Pain, 14*(4), 311–314.

Moritz, S., Hörmann, C., Schröder, J., Berger, T., Jacob, G., Meyer, B., . . Klein, J. (2014). Beyond words: Sensory properties of depressive thoughts. *Cognition and Emotion, 28*(6), 1047–1056.

Morriss, R. K., Wearden, A. J. F., & Battersby, L. (1997). The relation of sleep difficulties to fatigue, mood and disability in chronic fatigue syndrome. *Journal of Psychosomatic Research, 42*(6), 597–605.

Moya, H. (2009). Identities on paper: Constructing lives for people with intellectual disabilities in life story books. *Narrative Inquiry, 19*(1), 135–153.

Mundt, J. C., Marks, I. M., Shear, M. K., & Greist, J. M. (2002). The Work and Social Adjustment Scale: A simple measure of impairment in functioning. *The British Journal of Psychiatry, 180*(5), 461–464.

Murberg, T. A., Furze, G., & Bru, E. (2004). Avoidance coping styles predict mortality among patients with congestive heart failure: A 6-year follow-up study. *Personality and Individual Differences, 36*(4), 757–766.

Murray, H., Grey, N., Wild, J., Warnock-Parkes, E., Kerr, A., Clark, D. M., & Ehlers, A. (2020). Cognitive therapy for post-traumatic stress disorder following critical illness and intensive care unit admission. *The Cognitive Behaviour Therapist*, 1–36. Retrieved July 26, 2019, from www.nhs.uk/conditions/; www.healthylondon.org/wp-content/uploads/2017/11/IAPT-LTC-Full-Implementation-Guidance.pdf

Muse, K., McManus, F., Hackman, A., Williams, M., & Williams, M. (2010). Intrusive imagery in severe health anxiety: Prevalence, nature and links with memories and maintenance cycles. *Behaviour Research and Therapy, 48*(8), 792–798.

National Collaborating Centre for Mental Health. (2018). *The Improving Access to Psychological Therapies (IAPT) pathway for people with long-term physical health conditions and medically unexplained symptoms. Full implementation guidance.* London: National Collaborating Centre for Mental Health.

Neenan, M., & Dryden, W. (2013). *Life coaching: A cognitive behavioural approach.* Oxford: Routledge.

NICE. (2009). *Depression in adults with a chronic physical health problem: Recognition and management.* Clinical Guideline [CG91].

Nicholson, T. R., Aybek, S., Craig, T., Harris, T., Wojcik, W., David, A. S., & Kanaan, R. A. (2016). Life events and escape in conversion disorder. *Psychological Medicine, 46*(12), 2617–2626.

Nimnuan, C., Hotopf, M., & Wessely, S. (2001). Medically unexplained symptoms: An epidemiological study in seven specialities. *Journal of Psychosomatic Research, 51*(1), 361–367.

Nitter, A. K., Pripp, A. H., & Forseth, K. Ø. (2012). Are sleep problems and non-specific health complaints risk factors for chronic pain? A prospective population-based study with 17-year follow-up. *Scandinavian Journal of Pain, 3*(4), 210–217.

O'Brien, E. M., Waxenberg, L. B., Atchison, J. W., Gremillion, H. A., Staud, R. M., McCrae, C. S., & Robinson, M. E. (2010). Negative mood mediates the effect of poor sleep on pain among chronic pain patients. *The Clinical Journal of Pain, 26*(4), 310–319.

O'Connor, S. R., Tully, M. A., Ryan, B., Bleakley, C. M., Baxter, G. D., Bradley, J. M., & McDonough, S. M. (2015). Walking exercise for chronic musculoskeletal pain: Systematic review and meta-analysis. *Archives of Physical Medicine and Rehabilitation, 96*(4), 724–734.

Ost, L., & Sterner, U. (1987). Applied tension. A specific behavioral method for treatment of blood phobia. *Behaviour Research and Therapy, 25*(1), 25–29.

Oto, M., & Reuber, M. (2014). Psychogenic non-epileptic seizures: Aetiology, diagnosis, and management. *Advances in Psychiatric Treatment, 20*(1), 13–22.

Padesky, C. A. (2009). *Imagery in CBT.* Audio DVD. Centre for Cognitive Therapy.

Padesky, C. A. (2020). *Clinician's guide to CBT using mind over mood.* New York: Guilford Press.

Padesky, C. A., & Mooney, K. A. (2012). Strengths-based cognitive-behavioural therapy: A four-step model to build resilience. *Clinical Psychology and Psychotherapy, 19,* 283–290.

Panayiotou, G., Leonidou, C., Constantinou, E., Hart, J., Rinehart, K. L., Sy, J. T., & Björgvinsson, T. (2015). Do alexithymic individuals avoid their feelings? Experiential avoidance mediates the association between alexithymia, psychosomatic, and depressive symptoms in a community and a clinical sample. *Comprehensive Psychiatry, 56,* 206–216.

Papworth, M., & Marrinan, T. (2019). *Low intensity cognitive behaviour therapy* (2nd ed.). Los Angeles: Sage.

Pearson, J., Naselaris, T., Holmes, E., & Kosslin, S. (2015). Mental imagery: Functional mechanisms and clinical applications. *Trends in Cognitive Sciences, 19*(10), 590–602.

Pearson, M., Brewin, C. R., Rhodes, J., & McCarron, G. (2008). Frequency and nature of rumination in chronic depression: A preliminary study. *Cognitive Behaviour Therapy, 37,* 160–168.

Pelekasis, P., Matsouka, I., & Koumarionou, A. (2017). Progressive muscle relaxation as a supportive intervention for cancer patients undergoing chemotherapy: A systematic review. *Palliative and Supportive Care, 15*(4), 465–473.

Pendleton, D. A., & Boschner, S. (1980). Communication of medical information in general practice consultations as a function of patient's social class. *Social Science and Medicine*, *14*, 669–673.

Peters, S., Stanley, I., Rose, M., Kaney, S., & Salmon, P. (2002). A randomized controlled trial of group aerobic exercise in primary care patients with persistent, unexplained physical symptoms. *Family Practice*, *19*(6), 665–674.

Petersen, M. W., Schroder, A., Jorgensen, T., Ornbol, E., Meinertz Dantoft T, Eliasen M, et al. (2020). Irritable bowel, chronic widespread pain, chronic fatigue and related syndromes are prevalent and highly overlapping in the general population. *DanFunD Scientific Representation*, *10*(1), 3273.

Pollatos, O., & Gramann, K. (2011). Electrophysiological evidence of early processing deficits in alexithymia. *Biological Psychology*, *87*(1), 113–121.

Pourová, M., Klocek, A., Řiháček, T., & Čevelíček, M. (2020). Therapeutic change mechanisms in adults with medically unexplained physical symptoms: A systematic review. *Journal of Psychosomatic Research*, 110124.

Preece, D., Becerra, R., Allan, A., Robinson, K., & Dandy, J. (2017). Establishing the theoretical components of alexithymia via factor analysis: Introduction and validation of the attention-appraisal model of alexithymia. *Personality and Individual Differences*, *119*, 341–352.

Prochaska, J. O., & DiClemente, C. C. (1983). Stages and processes of self-change of smoking: Toward an integrative model of change. *Journal of Consulting and Clinical Psychology*, *51*(3), 390.

Pugh, M. (2018). Cognitive behavioural chairwork. *International Journal of Cognitive Therapy*, *11*(1), 100–116.

Read, S. A., Morton, T. A., & Ryan, M. K. (2015). Negotiating identity: A qualitative analysis of stigma and support seeking in individuals with cerebral palsy. *Disability and Rehabilitation*, *37*, 1162–1169.

Rethorst, C. D., Landers, D. M., Nagoshi, C. G., & Ross, J. T. D. (2010). Efficacy of exercise in reducing depressive symptoms across 5-HTTLPR genotypes. *Medicine and Science in Sports and Exercise*, 2141–2147.

Reuber, M., Pukrop, R., Bauer, J., Derfuss, R., & Elger, C. E. (2004). Multidimensional assessment of personality in patients with psychogenic non-epileptic seizures. *Journal of Neurology, Neurosurgery & Psychiatry*, *75*(5), 743–748.

Richards, D., Ekers, D., Macmillan, D., Taylor, R. S., Byford, S., Warren, F. C., et al. (2016). Cost and outcome of behavioural activation versus cognitive behavioural therapy for depression (COBRA): A randomised, controlled, non-inferiority trial. *The Lancet*, *388*(10047), 871–880.

Richards, D., & Whyte, M. (2009). *Reach out: National programme educator materials to support the delivery of training for psychological wellbeing practitioners delivering low intensity interventions* (2nd ed.). Gorleston, UK: Rethink.

Richards, D., & Whyte, M. (2011). *Reach out: National programme educator materials to support the delivery of training for psychological wellbeing practitioners delivering low intensity interventions* (3rd ed.). Gorleston, UK: Rethink.

Rief, W., Heuser, J., & Fichter, M. M. (1996). What does the Toronto Alexithymia Scale TAS-R measure? *Journal of Clinical Psychology*, *52*(4), 423–429.

Rief, W., Hiller, W., & Margraf, J. (1998). Cognitive aspects of hypochondriasis and the somatization syndrome. *Journal of Abnormal Psychology*, *107*(4), 587.

Riekert, K. A., Ockene, J. K., & Pbert, L. (2013). *The handbook of health behaviour change* (4th ed.). New York: Springer.

Rimes, K. A., Papadopoulos, A. S., Cleare, A. J., & Chalder, T. (2014). Cortisol output in adolescents with chronic fatigue syndrome: Pilot study on the comparison with healthy adolescents and change after cognitive behavioural guided self-help treatment. *Journal of Psychosomatic Research, 77*(5), 409–414.

Ritz, T., Meuret, A. E., & Simon, E. (2013). Cardiovascular activity in blood-injection-injury phobia during exposure: Evidence for diphasic response patterns?. *Behaviour Research and Therapy, 51*(8), 460–468.

Robichaud, M., & Dugas, M. J. (2015). *The generalized anxiety disorder workbook: A comprehensive CBT guide for coping with uncertainty, worry, and fear*. Oakland: New Harbinger Publications.

Robichaud, M., Koerner, N., & Dugas, M. J. (2019). *Cognitive behavioral treatment for generalized anxiety disorder: From science to practice*. Oxford: Routledge.

Roelofs, K., & Spinhoven, P. (2007). Trauma and medically unexplained symptoms: Towards an integration of cognitive and neuro-biological accounts. *Clinical Psychology Review, 27*(7), 798–820.

Rose, R., & Philpot, T. (2005). *The child's own story: Life story work with traumatized children*. London: Jessica Kingsley Publishers.

Rustad, J. K., David, D., & Currier, M. B. (2012). Cancer and post-traumatic stress disorder: Diagnosis, pathogenesis, and treatment considerations. *Palliative & Supportive Care, 10*(3), 213–223.

Ryan, T., & Walker, R. (2007). *Life story work: A practical guide to helping children understand their past*. London: British association for adoption and fostering.

Ryan, T., & Walker, R. (2016). *Life story work: How, what, why and when*. London: Coram BAAF.

Salkovskis, P. M. (1989). Chapter 7 'Somatic problems'. In K. Hawton, P. M. Salkovskis, J. Kirk, & D. M. Clark (Eds.), *Cognitive behavioural therapy for psychiatric problems: A practical guide*. Oxford: Oxford University Press.

Salkovskis, P. M., Rimes, K. A., & Warwick, H. M. C. (2002). The health anxiety inventory: Development and validation of scales for the measurement of health anxiety and hypochondriasis. *Psychological Medicine, 32*(5), 843.

Salkovskis, P. M., & Warwick, H. M. (1986). Morbid preoccupations, health anxiety and reassurance: A cognitive-behavioural approach to hypochondriasis. *Behaviour Research and Therapy, 24*(5), 597–602.

Samur, D., Tops, M., Schlinkert, C., Quirin, M., Cuijpers, P., & Koole, S. L. (2013). Four decades of research on alexithymia: Moving toward clinical applications. *Frontiers in Psychology, 4*, 861.

Sapolsky, R. M. (2004). *Why zebras don't get ulcers: The acclaimed guide to stress, stress-related diseases, and coping*. New York: Holt Paperbacks.

Schröder, A., Sharpe, M., & Fink, P. (2015). Medically unexplained symptom management. *The Lancet Psychiatry, 2*(7), 587–588.

Schwartz, G. E., & Beatty, J. (Eds.). (1977). *Biofeedback: Theory and research*. New York: Academic Press.

Scott, K. M., Hwang, I., Chiu, W. T., Kessler, R. C., Sampson, N. A., Angermeyer, M., . . . Florescu, S. (2010). Chronic physical conditions and their association with first onset of suicidal behavior in the world mental health surveys. *Psychosomatic Medicine, 72*(7), 712–719.

Sederer, L. I., Derman, M., Carruthers, J., & Wall, M. (2016). The New York state collaborative care initiative: 2012–2014. *Psychiatric Quarterly, 87*(1), 1–23.

Segal, Z. V., & Teasdale, J. (2018). *Mindfulness-based cognitive therapy for depression*. New York: Guilford Press.

Seligman, M. E., & Beagley, G. (1975). Learned helplessness in the rat. *Journal of Comparative and Physiological Psychology*, *88*(2), 534–541.

Seligman, M. E., & Csikszentmihalyi, M. (2014). Positive psychology: An introduction. In *Flow and the foundations of positive psychology* (pp. 279–298). Dordrecht: Springer.

Selmi, P. (1990). Computer-administered cognitive-behavioral therapy for depression. *American Journal of Psychiatry*, *147*(1), 51–56.

Sharpe, M., Stone, J., Hibberd, C., Warlow, C., Duncan, R., Coleman, R., . . . Matthews, K. (2010). Neurology out-patients with symptoms unexplained by disease: Illness beliefs and financial benefits predict 1-year outcome. *Psychological Medicine*, *40*(4), 689–698.

Simon, G., Gater, R., Kisely, S., & Piccinelli, M. (1996). Somatic symptoms of distress: An international primary care study. *Psychosomatic Medicine*, *58*(5), 481–488.

Skinner, B. F. (1955). *Science and human behavior*. New York: Simon and Schuster.

Skovenborg, E. L., & Schröder, A. (2014). Is physical disease missed in patients with medically unexplained symptoms? A long-term follow-up of 120 patients diagnosed with bodily distress syndrome. *General Hospital Psychiatry*, *36*(1), 38–45.

Spek, V., Nyklicek, I., Smita, N., Cuijpers, P., Riper, H., Keyzer, J., & Pop, V. (2007). Internet-based cognitive behavioural therapy for subthreshold depression in people over 50 years old: A randomised controlled clinical trial. *Psychological Medicine*, *37*(12), 1797–1806.

Spence, M. J., Moss-Morris, R., Spence, M. J., & Moss-Morris, R. (2007). The cognitive behavioural model of irritable bowel syndrome: A prospective investigation of patients with gastroenteritis. *Gut*, *56*(8), 1066–1071.

Spitzer, R. L., Kroenke, K., Williams, J. B., & Löwe, B. (2006). A brief measure for assessing generalized anxiety disorder: The GAD-7. *Archives of Internal Medicine*, *166*(10), 1092–1097.

St Claire, L., & Clucas, C. (2012). In sickness and in health: Influences of social categorizations on health-related outcomes, In J. Jetten, C. Haslam, & S. A. Haslam (Eds.), *The social cure: Identity, health and well-being* (pp. 75–95). Hove, UK: Psychology Press.

Steinbrecher, N., & Hiller, W. (2011). Course and prediction of somatoform disorder and medically unexplained symptoms in primary care. *General Hospital Psychiatry*, *33*(4), 318–326.

Stone, J., Sharpe, M., Rothwell, P. M., & Warlow, C. P. (2003). The 12-year prognosis of unilateral functional weakness and sensory disturbance. *Journal of Neurology, Neurosurgery & Psychiatry*, *74*(5), 591–596.

Susko, M. (1994). Caseness and narrative – contrasting approaches to people who are psychiatrically labeled. *Journal of Mind and Behaviour*, *15*(1–2), 87–112.

Tang, T. Z., DeRubeis, R. J., Beberman, R., & Pham, T. (2005). Cognitive changes, critical sessions, and sudden gains in cognitive-behavioral therapy for depression. *Journal of Consulting and Clinical Psychology*, *73*(1), 168–172.

Taylor, G. J., Ryan, D., & Bagby, M. (1985). Toward the development of a new self-report alexithymia scale. *Psychotherapy and Psychosomatics*, *44*(4), 191–199.

Taylor, R. (2006). *Cognitive behavioural therapy for chronic illness and disability*. New York: Springer.

Thomas, S. A., Drummond, A. E., Lincoln, N. B., Palmer, R. L., das Nair, R., Latimer, N. R., . . Topcu, G. (2019). Behavioural activation therapy for post-stroke depression: The BEADS feasibility RCT. *Health Technology Assessment (Winchester, England)*, *23*(47), 1–176.

Tominaga, T., Choi, H., Nagoshi, Y., Wada, Y., & Fukui, K. (2014). Relationship between alexithymia and coping strategies in patients with somatoform disorder. *Neuropsychiatric Disease and Treatment, 10*, 55.

Tully, P. J., Sardinha, A., & Nardi, A. E. (2017). A new CBT model of panic attack treatment in comorbid heart diseases (PATCHD): How to calm an anxious heart and mind. *Cognitive and Behavioral Practice, 24*(3), 329–341.

Twohig, M. P., & Levin, M. E. (2017). Acceptance and commitment therapy as a treatment for anxiety and depression: A review. *Psychiatric Clinics, 40*(4), 751–770.

Tyrer, H. (2013). *Tackling health anxiety: A CBT handbook.* London: RCP publications.

Tyrer, P., Cooper, S., Salkovskis, P., Tyrer, H., Crawford, M., Byford, S., . . . Murphy, D. (2014). Clinical and cost-effectiveness of cognitive behaviour therapy for health anxiety in medical patients: A multicentre randomised controlled trial. *The Lancet, 383*(9913), 219–225.

Tyrer, P., Cooper, S., Tyrer, H., Salkovskis, P., Crawford, M., Green, J., . . . Byford, S. (2011). CHAMP: Cognitive behaviour therapy for health anxiety in medical patients, a randomised controlled trial. *BMC Psychiatry, 11*(1), 99.

Tyrer, P., Salkovskis, P., Tyrer, H., Wang, D., Crawford, M. J., Dupont, S., . . . Bhogal, S. (2017). Cognitive–behaviour therapy for health anxiety in medical patients (CHAMP): A randomised controlled trial with outcomes to 5 years. *Health Technology Assessment, 21*(50), 1–58.

Uphoff, E., Pires, M., Barbui, C., Barua, D., Churchill, R., Cristofalo, D., . . Siddiqi, N. (2020). Behavioural activation therapy for depression in adults with non-communicable diseases (review). *Cochrane Database of Systematic Reviews 2020*, (8). Art. No.: CD013461.

Uslan, D. (2003). Rehabilitation counselling. In L. A. Jason, P. A. Fennell, & R. R. Taylor (Eds.), *Handbook of chronic fatigue syndrome.* New York: Wiley.

Van Dessel, N., Den Boeft, M., van der Wouden, J. C., Kleinstaeuber, M., Leone, S. S., Terluin, B., . . . van Marwijk, H. (2014). Non-pharmacological interventions for somatoform disorders and medically unexplained physical symptoms (MUPS) in adults. *Cochrane Database of Systematic Reviews*, (11).

Van Dijk, S. D. M., Hanssen, D., Naarding, P., Lucassen, P. L. B. J., Comijs, H., & Voshaar, R. O. (2016). Big Five personality traits and medically unexplained symptoms in later life. *European Psychiatry, 38*, 23–30.

Van Egmond, J. J. (2003). Multiple meanings of secondary gain. *The American Journal of Psychoanalysis, 63*(2), 137–147.

Van Egmond, J. J., & Kummeling, I. (2002). A blind spot for secondary gain affecting therapy outcomes. *European Psychiatry, 17*(1), 46–54.

Veale, D., & Willson, R. (2009). *Overcoming health anxiety: A self-help guide using cognitive behavioural techniques.* London: Hachette UK.

Victor, P., Krug, I., Vehoff, C., Lyons, N., & Willutzki, U. (2018). Strengths-based CBT: Internet-based versus face-to-face therapy in a randomized controlled trial. *Journal of Depression and Anxiety, 7*, 301.

Vilchinsky, N., Ginzburg, K., Fait, K., & Foa, E. B. (2017). Cardiac-disease-induced PTSD (CDI-PTSD): A systematic review. *Clinical Psychology Review, 55*, 92–106.

Vcgele, C., Coles, J., Wardle, J., & Steptoe, A. (2003). Psychophysiologic effects of applied tension on the emotional fainting response to blood and injury. *Behaviour Research and Therapy, 41*(2), 139–155.

Vlaeyen, J. W., & Linton, S. J. (2000). Fear-avoidance and its consequences in chronic musculoskeletal pain: A state of the art. *Pain, 85*(3), 317–332.

Wakefield, J. R., Bickley, S., & Sani, F. (2013). The effects of identification with a support group on the mental health of people with multiple sclerosis. *Journal of Psychosomatic Research, 74*(5), 420–426.

Wells, A., & Hackmann, A. (1993). Imagery and core beliefs in health anxiety: Content and origins. *Behavioural and Cognitive Psychotherapy, 21*(3), 265–273.

Wheatley, J., Brewin, C. J., Patel, T., Hackman, A., Wells, A., Fisher, P., & Myers, S. (2007). I'll believe it when I see it: Imagery rescripting of intrusive sensory memories in depression. *Journal of Behavioural Therapy and Experimental Psychiatry, 38*(4), 371–385.

Wheatley, J., & Hackmann, A. (2011). Using imagery rescripting to treat major depression: Theory and practice. *Cognitive and Behavioral Practice, 18*(4), 444–453.

Whitaker, K. L., Brewin, C. R., & Watson, M. (2010). Imagery rescripting for psychological disorder following cancer: A case study. *British Journal of Health Psychology, 15*, 41–50.

WHO (2017). *World health statistics 2017: Monitoring health for the sustainable development goals* (SDGs). Geneva: WHO.

Whooley, M. A., Avins, A. L., Miranda, J., & Browner, W. S. (1997). Case-finding instruments for depression. Two questions are as good as many. *Journal of General Internal Medicine, 12*, 439–445.

Wileman, L., May, C., & Chew-Graham, C. A. (2002). Medically unexplained symptoms and the problem of power in the primary care consultation: A qualitative study. *Family Practice, 19*(2), 178–182.

Wilkinson, M., Venning, A., Redpath, P., Ly, M., Brown, S., & Battersby, M. (2019). Can low intensity cognitive behavioural therapy for non-cardiac chest pain presentations to an emergency department be efficacious? A pilot study. *Australian Psychologist, 54*(6), 494–501.

Williams, A. D., Blackwell, S. E., Mackenzie, A., Holmes, E. A., & Andrews, G. (2013). Combining imagination and reason in the treatment of depression: A randomized controlled trial of internet-based cognitive-bias modification and internet-CBT for depression. *Journal of Consulting and Clinical Psychology, 81*(5), 793.

Williams, C., & Chellingsworth, M. (2010). *CBT: A clinician's guide to using the five areas approach*. London: Hodder Arnold.

Wooley, S. C., Blackwell, B., & Winget, C. (1978). A learning theory model of chronic illness behavior: Theory, treatment, and research. *Psychosomatic Medicine, 40*(5), 379–401.

Woolfolk, R. L., & Allen, L. A. (2007). *Treating somatization: A cognitive behavioural approach*. New York: Guilford Press.

Wroe, A. L., Rennie, E. W., Gibbons, S., Hassy, A., & Chapman, J. (2015). IAPT and long-term medical conditions: What can we offer? *Behavioural and Cognitive Psychotherapy, 43*, 415–425.

Wroe, A. L, Rennie, E. W., Sollesse, S., Chapman, J., & Hassy, J. (2018). Is cognitive behavioural therapy focusing on depression and anxiety effective for people with long-term physical health conditions? A controlled trial in the context of type 2 diabetes mellitus. *Behavioural and Cognitive Psychotherapy, 46*(2), 129–147.

Xiong, J., Lipsitz, O., Nasri, F., Lui, L. M., Gill, H., Phan, L., . . . McIntyre, R. S. (2020). Impact of COVID-19 pandemic on mental health in the general population: A systematic review. *Journal of Affective Disorders, 277*, 55–64.

Yon, K., Habermann, S., Rosenthal, J., Walters, K. R., Nettleton, S., Warner, A., & Busze-
    wicz, M. (2017). Improving teaching about medically unexplained symptoms for newly
    qualified doctors in the UK: Findings from a questionnaire survey and expert workshop.
    *BMJ Open, 7*(4)

Young, A., & Rodriguez, K. (2006). The role of narrative in discussing end-of-life care:
    Eliciting values and goals from text, context and subtext. *Health Communication, 19*(1),
    49–59.

# Index

Note: Page numbers in *italics* indicate a figure and page numbers in **bold** indicate a table on the corresponding page.